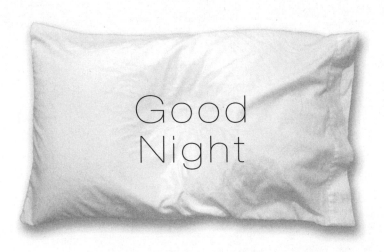

Good
Night

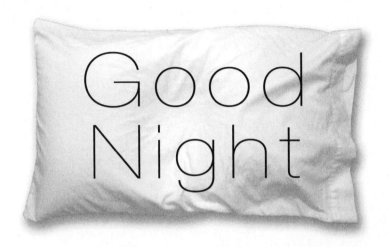

Good Night

The Sleep Doctor's 4-Week Program to Better Sleep and Better Health

MICHAEL BREUS, Ph.D.

DUTTON

DUTTON
Published by Penguin Group (USA) Inc.
375 Hudson Street, New York, New York 10014, U.S.A.
Penguin Group (Canada), 90 Eglinton Avenue East, Suite 700, Toronto, Ontario M4P 2Y3, Canada
(a division of Pearson Penguin Canada Inc.); Penguin Books Ltd, 80 Strand, London WC2R 0RL,
England; Penguin Ireland, 25 St Stephen's Green, Dublin 2, Ireland (a division of Penguin Books
Ltd); Penguin Group (Australia), 250 Camberwell Road, Camberwell, Victoria 3124, Australia (a
division of Pearson Australia Group Pty Ltd); Penguin Books India Pvt Ltd, 11 Community Centre,
Panchsheel Park, New Delhi – 110 017, India; Penguin Group (NZ), cnr Airborne and Rosedale
Roads, Albany, Auckland 1310, New Zealand (a division of Pearson New Zealand Ltd); Penguin
Books (South Africa) (Pty) Ltd, 24 Sturdee Avenue, Rosebank, Johannesburg 2196, South Africa

Penguin Books Ltd, Registered Offices: 80 Strand, London WC2R 0RL, England

Published by Dutton, a member of Penguin Group (USA) Inc.

First printing, September 2006
10 9 8 7 6 5 4 3 2 1

 REGISTERED TRADEMARK — MARCA REGISTRADA

LIBRARY OF CONGRESS CATALOGING-IN-PUBLICATION DATA
Breus, Michael.
    Good night : the sleep doctor's 4-week program to better sleep and better health /
Michael Breus.—1st ed.
        p.   cm.
ISBN 0-525-94979-8 (hardcover)
1. Sleep—Health aspects.   I. Title.
RA786.B74 2006
613.7'94—dc22   2006015147

Printed in the United States of America
Set in Goudy
Photograph by Jae Song
Designed by Eve L. Kirch

While the author has made every effort to provide accurate telephone numbers and Internet addresses at the time of publication, neither the publisher nor the author assumes any responsibility for
errors, or for changes that occur after publication. Further, the publisher does not have any control
over and does not assume any responsibility for author or third-party Web sites or their content.

To Lauren, for listening to me answer the same questions over and over. For sleeping with the TV on. For trying every new sleep gadget I can find. For giving me the gift of the two best children in the world. For all of your love and support, I could never have done this without you.

CONTENTS

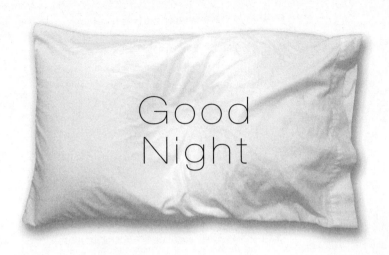

Good
Night

INTRODUCTION:
A VITAL SIGN OF HEALTH

Nothing is more frustrating than getting a bad night's sleep and feeling tired, cranky, and older the next day . . . and the day after that. It's perfectly normal to feel fatigue once in a while. But when we experience long-term exhaustion, disappointment in our productivity, illness, weight gain, and general feelings of depression and dissatisfaction with life, few of us stop to consider the one thing that can alleviate, if not prevent, all that: sleep. This is your guide to getting supreme sleep. This is your personal manual for finding sound sleep night after night to the best of your ability. Sleep problems are, after all, estimated to be the number one health issue in the United States.

Many people are living like zombies, sacrificing sleep to meet waking deadlines and turning to drugs and stimulants to stay awake, or drugs and depressants to fall asleep and remain that way until the morning alarm rings. A record 43 million prescriptions for sleeping pills were written by U.S. doctors in 2005, and by 2010 it's been estimated that the pharmaceutical industry will be reaping at least $5 billion a year from such sales. Why? Because people want better sleep. In pursuit of youth and beauty, a popular option is to resort to invasive and risky cosmetic procedures, plus pills and potions touted to make one look and feel younger. Current medicine and the media make these procedures and "cosmeceuticals" look easy and safe. And I am here to tell you these alternatives are not always easy and effective, nor are they necessarily cheap and safe. Popular diets and weight-loss pills can't always guarantee you'll lose ten pounds forever. Products that claim to boost our energy levels have generated such a market that we now have energy drinks that sell to everyone from teenagers to adults (some people even mix these with alcohol). Our society's hunger (and thirst) for more energy and more time seems to grow every day.

If you're reading this book because you have a known sleep disorder or are pretty sure you do, then this may only be a program to use in conjunction with working with a sleep specialist. But if you know you've got a problem and you can't put sleep at the bottom of your list of priorities anymore, you've come to the right place. I've got the prescription for rejuvenating your mind and body, improving your sex life, increasing your energy reserves and vitality, and helping you lose weight and keep it off. This won't require anything more than a commitment to getting restful, sound sleep, and the programs presented in this book will show you how to achieve that goal. It will change the way you think. It will enhance the way you live.

A Magical Transformation

I once had a woman come to me on a referral from her best friend, Susan W., whom I'd treated just two months prior. Nancy P. was thirty-two years old. Looking very animated and anxious to tell her story, she was quick to start talking. I'd heard a version of her story many times before:

> I was having lunch with my best friend the other day. We've known each other since grade school and have been very close since high school. Over the years we've shared a lot in common. We both got married around the same time, and then we were pregnant with our second children the same year. We get together a lot and always seem to talk about the hardships of trying to fit everything in—you know, mixing being a parent, a wife, and a worker outside the home. It's hard.
>
> Well, the other day was the first time I'd seen Susan in about a month. And I was literally shocked by her appearance. Her skin looked so . . . fresh—as if she'd just had some kind of major dermatological treatment or even seen a cosmetic surgeon. Her face was vibrant, colorful, I don't know

how to describe it . . . alive, I guess. I mean, now she looks several years younger than me—and we're both the same age! I know Susan complained a few months ago that she'd been having a lot of sleep problems, and I knew ex-actly what she was talking about. But I didn't think she'd actually do anything about it. Or that it would change so much about her so quickly. She looks so damn good! She's lost weight, too, and says that she now has the energy to ex-ercise. She even mentioned something about her sex life!

Anyway, she said it was all you. I've never been to a sleep doctor and I find it hard to believe sleep can do so much to a person. But I've tried every-thing and nothing has worked. Susan and I used to be equals, and now I feel left behind. I don't want to look fifty when I'm not even forty yet. Dr. Breus, please help me, too. I didn't realize how bad I looked until I went home and locked myself in the bathroom in front of the mirror. . . .

Nancy went on to explain more about her own situation, and I per-formed my evaluation to determine what kind of suggestions I needed to make. Nancy's story was very typical of many of the women who come see me. She'd been experiencing chronic exhaustion from balancing the demands of motherhood and work for quite some time, and she said that it wasn't until she turned thirty that her energy level really began to di-minish. She constantly found herself staying up late at night to finish up chores and get ready for the next day. There was never a dull moment on weekends, either. When I asked her how long she'd been having sleep problems, she surprised herself, realizing that she hadn't had a long period of restful sleep in about five years—before she began having chil-dren. This is also very typical of the patients I see: They are not fully aware of the extent to which sleep deprivation has truly affected how they look and feel on a daily basis. I prompt them with a series of ques-tions that usually ends with their saying, "Oh my gosh, you're right," or, "How come it took me this long to realize what my sleep problems are doing to me?" They are also eager to know if the damage is reversible or if they're stuck with how they've aged up until now. Two very com-monly asked questions are, "Can I turn back my clock with sleep? Can I take back all that sleep debt?" And that's when I smile reassuringly.

I went through a full analysis of Nancy and we noted several things: Her skin was uncharacteristically pale and washed out; she'd failed every diet in attempts to lose the weight that came with pregnancy, and was now about twenty pounds overweight. When I questioned her sex life, she openly admitted that it hadn't returned to its pre-children status. "Mark has begun to complain about the 'distance' between us," she said. "He says I'm not the same person anymore. I'm moody, irritable, unavailable. I say I'm tired all the time, because I am. And what really hurt is when he said that I've 'let myself go.'" This troubled Nancy greatly. I glimpsed a few tears when she began to talk about this aspect to her marriage.

"It's okay," I said. "I have a solution."

I started Nancy on a plan that got her sleep life in order. As it turned out, her problems were worse than her friend's. She had terrible eating habits, including a serious addiction to caffeinated soda in the morning and coffee in the late afternoon; she hated the thought of exercise; and she had a husband who snored and thrashed about the bed at night so badly that it often kept her up or moved her into the den. So she had a lot to accomplish, but she was ready and willing to take action.

Three weeks after Nancy started to make small changes to her lifestyle—all of which you'll come to learn about in this book—I got a call from her. I had asked her to check in with me at this juncture. Right away I knew she had good news to share.

"Dr. Breus! It's working! I know that it's only been a few weeks, but I am amazed at what's happening. I feel so much better and I've already lost four pounds."

"That's wonderful, Nancy. What's been the hardest part to staying on your program?"

"Curbing the caffeine and doing exercise is tough, but I'm feeling so good that it's all worth it. I haven't felt this energetic in years, and my husband wants to come see you now. I saw Susan today, and 'Wow' was all she could say. . . ."

Results like this are exactly why I'm in this specialty. It's incredibly exciting for me to watch someone follow my advice and see immediate, long-lasting results. Nancy eventually met her goals: She lost the extra weight, changed her skin tone and appearance for the better, and found the energy to begin a realistic exercise regimen. Her husband was so delightfully surprised by her transformation that he, too, paid me a visit and I began treating them as a couple. It didn't take long for them to rediscover their relationship in the bedroom. Nancy called it the "second honeymoon." Further down the road, her husband managed to modify his own sleep habits, which shed his extra (thirty!) pounds and eliminated his snoring completely.

I repeat: The above story is not atypical. I see it all the time. Day in and day out I see patients with one underlying problem—sleep—that contributes enormously to a host of other problems in their lives, including physical, psychological, *and* interpersonal. What Susan, Nancy, and Nancy's husband discovered is what thousands of my patients have already discovered and what I want you to find: the fountain of youth and beauty in sleep.

I know that it's hard for some of my patients to make serious changes in their lives, but look what happens: They end up looking and feeling younger. Their friends and family notice. They become role models for others to transform themselves. I believe those changes do more for their quality of life than any pill, therapist, or cosmetic surgery can do. I feel like I've saved more marriages in my work than I would have as a marital therapist. I've been fortunate enough to witness grown men and women cry in my office as they share their gratitude for my work and how it has enhanced their lives, ended divorce proceedings, and revitalized their marriages. I find it enjoyable when I'm at a cocktail or dinner party and someone approaches me from across the room with a curious, determined look on his or her face and asks, "I hear you're a sleep doctor? Is that true?" He or she always wants to hear about my work, and how I became a sleep doctor. Sleep, as I've found, is a topic that fascinates everybody. I'm just a lucky guy.

My Road to Becoming a Sleep Doc

I never intended to become a sleep specialist. I was working toward my Ph.D. in psychology and had begun my internship program at the University of Mississippi Medical Center, where I originally set out to specialize in eating disorders in athletes. But, to my dismay, that particular program was full. So I then matriculated in the university's sleep program thinking that I'd switch into the eating disorder program as soon as possible.

That, of course, didn't happen. By the end of the first week in the sleep clinic, I knew I had found my calling in clinical sleep medicine. I couldn't find any other specialty in which I could help someone so quickly and dramatically. I could change a person's life in forty-eight hours where it may take years to do the same with traditional methods in conventional therapy. Working as a team with other professionals, including physicians, pulmonologists, neurologists, and psychiatrists, among others, has made for a uniquely thrilling career. There's never a dull day.

Over the years I've made it my mission to bring awareness of sleep to the center of popular medicine and change the way everyone—physicians and the public—views sleep. You might already be familiar with my advice, but not necessarily know it. I've been working hard to communicate sleep awareness to you. You deserve to know. Unfortunately, your family doctor or general practitioner never learned it in school.

If you've been a passenger on a major airline you may have encountered my tips on in-flight videos or seen me on CNN's Airport Network. Or perhaps you've logged on to WebMD.com and entered its message board, blog, video archive, or read my column in its magazine. That's where I am the designated health expert specializing in sleep and enjoy hearing about and responding to the thousands of complaints people have about their problems with sleep. If you've recently stayed in a Crowne Plaza hotel, you might also have come across our Sleep Advantage® program. I'm doing what I can to transform society one person at a time. I want to bring an end to your thinking that sleep deprivation is a sad fact of life, and get you to recognize that sleep is the number one missing ingredient to living leaner, looking younger, and feeling sexier.

We've come a long way in understanding how our bodies age and what accelerates the aging process. Breakthrough science is now showing us how and why sleep affects how we look, feel, and function. Health problems such as obesity, diabetes, hypertension, depression, and even chronic pain are related to the amount and quality of a person's sleep. It also has strong ties to healthy pregnancies. Aside from what science tells us, it doesn't take a genius to know that sleep shapes every facet of our lives. If it didn't, we probably wouldn't spend about a third of our lives doing it. Sleep has a direct impact on how well we work, relate to other people, accomplish goals, rate our sense of well-being, and avoid the onset of age-related disease. But here's the problem:

According to the National Institutes of Health, at least 70 million Americans have sleep problems for a few days or for several weeks or longer, while 40 million suffer for longer periods of time. Because of sleep problems, millions do not get enough sleep to function at their best during their waking hours. A good number of those people also report that sleep problems interfere with daily activities a few days or more a month. Over a lifetime, that can be a monstrous amount of wasted time.

I see a wide variety of sleep-deprived people in my practice, from those with serious sleep disorders to those who just need to make a few minor changes to their behavioral patterns and nighttime habits to look and feel years younger within a short period of time—sometimes within just a few days. Although I cover the topic of sleep disorders briefly and give you some guidance in determining whether you do, in fact, have a sleep disorder that requires medical attention, I am writing this book primarily for the people whose sleep problems can be solved through a few lifestyle modifications. If sleep doesn't come easily to you, or you call yourself an insomniac and have trouble sleeping soundly through the night, chances are this book can rescue your sleep and lessen, if not totally eradicate, your problems.

In This Book

This book is not about giving up coffee and alcohol entirely, locking yourself in your bedroom once the clock hits 9 P.M., or drastically changing your lifestyle to the point you don't act (or feel) like yourself anymore. It's about making subtle modifications over time that are practical and reasonable. It's about manipulating a free asset in your life—sleep—to strike a balance between accomplishing all that you want in life while looking your best and defying the laws of aging. All too often we tend to sacrifice sleep in our daily quest for success. We pay for that sacrifice in an accelerated aging process, in our moods and relationships with other people, and in our own sense of personal satisfaction.

You'll learn an abundance of information in this book, and it won't be just about the science behind sleep in simple terms. (In fact, I won't be rehashing all the textbook-like information on sleep that you can surely find elsewhere. I'll summarize briefly what I think you need to know and will go into greater depth on topics that are either extremely important or that present new information. I didn't write this book so you can become a lecturing sleep expert on the subject per se; I wrote it so you can use what we know in the science of sleep to then make smart decisions about your sleep habits. This book is about *applying* the science to your life in the real world rather than understanding all that science.)

The self-evaluations I have created will get you to take an honest look at yourself and tune in to the internal workings of your body in relation to your personal world. You'll begin to understand how the body contains amazing self-preservation mechanisms (i.e., resources for looking and feeling younger) if you just let it get the quality sleep it craves. I hope that with the programs and suggestions made in this book, you'll come to rely on the power of well-balanced sleep to live longer and better rather than using drugs to help you sleep and stimulants to keep you awake. I'll teach you how to create the ideal sleep environment, calculate your optimal sleep requirements, incorporate naps into your day, cope with a partner's sleep behavior, as well as deal with problems from insomnia to your body's cyclical, rhythmic changes that affect sleep. I'll also show you where you need to go if the tests in this book lead you to believe you have a true sleep disorder.

This book is divided into four parts. At the beginning of the book, you'll be taken through a series of questionnaires and subsequent Action Plans that offer quick-fix solutions and can help you break bad habits that profoundly affect your sleep. I'll go through the six main thieves of sleep and teach you how to conquer them starting today. Then, we'll take a departure from the self-evaluations and mini-programs to learn the latest information on sleep in four categories: weight control, cosmetics, sex, and exercise. You'll wonder why no one told you this before, and why your doctor never asks you about your sleep habits in detail. How long has science known this? Well, to be honest, much of our knowledge about how sleep affects our body's machinery—from the inner workings of our brain and vital organs to our metabolism, ability to lose weight, sexual vigor, and overall health—is pretty new. We only recently discovered, for example, how sleep deprivation is linked to weight gain. I've put all the cutting-edge data into a usable form that you can apply to your life. I've broken down the science and crafted formulas that stem not only from the science, but from my years of clinical experience.

In the third part of this book, you'll have the opportunity to go on a 28-night program that takes you day by day (or night by night) through modifying your life around sleep. If you've tried to apply general tips for getting better sleep in the past without long-term success, this program might be your answer. Getting on a regimented plan that takes you day by day with specific goals and instructions can make a huge difference. It can condition you slowly over time to being a better sleeper without having to continually worry about sleep and fight against the inability to sleep well. My step-by-step program will capture lost sleep, shift your mindset so you welcome sleep naturally every night, and most importantly, it can help you begin to reach those prized goals in just twenty-eight nights: total weight management, all-natural beauty, energy for exercise and top performance, and a better sex life.

You'll start by finding your "number"—the perfect number of hours you need to feel rested and rejuvenated the next day—and then progress through a monthlong process of developing and mastering your sleep habits so they support a restful night's sleep at home and away. In the last part of the book, you'll pick up some tips for getting a good night's rest when you're not as much in control of your schedule as you'd like. I'll help frequent travelers stick to a program, I'll provide some guidance for shift workers, and I'll weigh in on sleep aids and prescription medications. The market is teeming with supplements, drugs, and remedies that promise you better sleep. Do any of these have merit? I'll discern the facts from fiction. Together we'll find what factors might be interfering with your sleep and together we'll try to conquer them.

I encourage you to visit my Web site at www.soundsleepsolutions.com, where you can access up-to-date information, links to excellent resources and sleep centers, and virtual guidance in performing simple bedtime stretches. You'll also be able to download portions of my relaxation/meditation CD for free and visit a store that offers other tools and products that will aid you in your journey to sound sleep. I welcome your feedback and personal stories. From the site you'll be able to e-mail me questions or particular problems you have along the way. I'll post answers to all the popular questions.

Setting Goals and Managing Expectations

A good night's sleep is now your top health priority. You're about to embark on a journey that will attempt to target your biggest problems when it comes to sleep, and then treat them. First, understand that not everyone will have the same issues or respond to the same recommenda-tions. Every reader comes to this book with a different set of problems and personal history—including medical, physical, emotional, and even philosophical—in how he or she approaches life in general. You'll be performing a lot of self-examinations to come to terms with your own particular situation, from which you can then formulate a plan of action.

To get the most out of this book's Action Plans and 28-night program, I want you to treat your sleep like a business. Set some goals right from the start and do your best to manage your expectations along the way as you would any important project at work. As you become an informed and mindful sleep analyst and self-counselor, you'll know which goals to set. And, like any serious lifestyle change to become healthier, leaner, and more alive, my program requires a commitment on your part. You'll need patience, a willingness to make some difficult alterations in your current way of living, as well as the dreaded D word: discipline. I'll ask you to scrutinize your life honestly and critically. I'll ask that you keep a sleep diary, a template of which is provided in Appendix A. No one else has to see what you record. The more open-minded you are to testing new methods and experimenting with various sleep-promoting habits in my program, the better chance you have at finding sound sleep . . . forever.

As you set your goals and manage your expectations, it's good to con-sider any obstacles you have that place you in a "special circumstances" category. For example, if you're a parent with a newborn in the home, you'll face added challenges and might have to accept less-than-perfect sleep during this time period. The same goes for people with medical conditions for which their necessary medications affect sleep, or the condition itself impacts their sleep. If you're a perimenopausal or meno-pausal woman, you have your own set of issues to contend with. Those going through acutely stressful periods due to financial struggles, marital strife, or other family troubles will also bear certain challenges. If you have lost someone special in your life, sleep may be elusive, but making sure you have proper sleep habits when it returns is important. Few peo-ple's lives are "perfect" at any given time. Nonetheless, everyone can still benefit enormously from this program; everyone's individual expectations, however, will be different. If you succeed in implementing the recommendations in this book, you'll likely notice a difference in how you look and feel regardless of your special circumstance. Be as persistent and committed as you can, and you will experience a positive change in the quality of your sleep no matter what.

The link between sleep and quality of life sprang out from the pages of a report released by the National Sleep Foundation in its annual poll called "Sleep in America." According to its 2005 landmark poll, which covered both men and women, 75 percent of us have symptoms of a sleep problem on a regular basis, such as waking a lot during the night, or snoring, but most of us ignore the signs and few of us think we actually have a sleep problem. A quarter of us admit that sleep problems have some impact on our daily lives. Only a handful of us ever takes any steps to improve our sleep. And about two in ten say that if we had a sleep problem we'd assume it would go away and we would take no action.

Throughout this book, I want you to keep one truth in mind: Getting high-quality sleep is a vital sign of health. Sleep is a necessity—not a luxury.

Think of this experience as an investment in yourself that returns years of health and happiness to you—a superior quality of life. There are no risks involved, no deleterious consequences, no major costs to bear. Only a new you to embrace.

Think of this as a health and beauty book that puts sleep at the top of the list of things to do.

Get ready to experience incredible results.

What makes you happy? Sleep. Sleep quality has a greater influence on the ability to enjoy your day than household income and even marital status. In 2004 researchers at Princeton and the University of Michigan used the Day Reconstruction Method (DRM)—a way of measuring how happy people feel at a given time—to analyze how 909 women actually spend their time and how they experience their various activities. **They found that an extra hour of sleep had more of an impact on how the participants felt throughout the day than earning more money a year. Their findings landed in the journal *Science* in December 2004.**

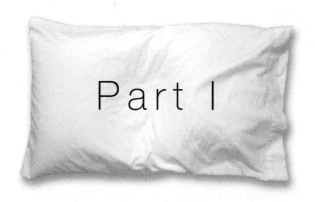

Part I

Quick-Fix
Sleep Solutions

CHAPTER 1

How Sleep Deprived Are You, and What Does That Mean?

Early in my career, I entered an exam room in our clinic prepared to do an initial office evaluation of a new patient. When I caught sight of a man with a gun, I knew this was going to be interesting. I did my best to appear professional and at ease, but I was a bit nervous. As I sat down I introduced myself and started asking questions. The man was in his early fifties, and he explained that he was with the GBI, short for Georgia Bureau of Investigation. He had been given a desk job about a year earlier . . . and the desk job was making him crazy.

"What happened?" I asked.

"I fell asleep on stake-outs and in meetings. My boss thought I had spent too much time in the field and that I needed to be put out to pasture."

Once we started talking I realized he exhibited several signs and symptoms of obstructive sleep apnea. To start, he was severely overweight. He said he snored so loudly that his wife slept in a different bedroom. "I fly off the handle all the time and get angry at little things that never really bothered me before," he explained.

"Are you sleepy during the day?" I asked.

"Doc, I am so sleepy during the day that I fall asleep at my desk. My colleagues like to throw things at me—and drop books near my head—in the hopes of waking me up."

"And what about at nighttime? Do you have trouble staying asleep through the night?"

His answer was yes, and he added that he always fell asleep in the living room recliner. He'd awaken with a dry mouth and a headache. He had no energy. The cycle would repeat itself almost every day.

My first course of action was to order a sleep study (called a polysomnogram), which proved my instincts correct: He had a bad case of apnea, a sleep disorder that affects the quality and ability to sleep soundly. A person with sleep apnea literally stops breathing until the brain awakens the body to the problem and the person gasps for air, then returns to normal breathing or snoring until the cycle begins again. This man's apnea was so miserable that his breathing halted more than seventy times an hour, and hundreds of times a night. His oxygen levels were so low at night that he could have suffered a stroke; his heart had to work overtime by slowing down when he stopped breathing and then revving back up quickly to wake him for a breath of air. His situation was no different from that of 50 percent of my patients.

With the help of my colleagues in the office I suggested that the man be placed on a CPAP machine—which stands for Continuous Positive Airway Pressure—a device that keeps a small stream of air blowing into the airways to prevent the throat from collapsing all night long and blocking the breath's passageway. This maintains regular breathing.

When he woke the morning after the sleep study, he could not believe how much better he felt. He took a CPAP machine home, and I asked that he get at least seven hours of sleep a night. I would see him again in a month.

When he returned a month later, his wife accompanied him. As soon as I introduced myself she sprang up and gave me the biggest hug anyone at the clinic had ever given me. She began to cry, recalling that since they had been sleeping apart, and since he had been so bad-tempered, she had gone to a lawyer and commenced divorce proceedings. She had planned on serving him the papers, but was waiting to see what kind of difference our treatment would make. I looked over at my patient, a man of modest emotion but obvious gratitude. He reached into his pocket and pulled out his card. He scribbled a number on the back of it and said, "Doc, if you are ever in trouble, call this number . . . and you won't be."

I keep the card in a very safe place.

As the couple was leaving, holding hands, the wife turned and handed me the divorce papers, saying, "I don't think I will be needing these."

Did you read the Introduction? If you haven't, go back and read it. I know, I don't always read intros, either. But this one explains several essential aspects to this book, and I want to make sure you know what you're getting into. If you're all ready to go, then read on to discover the wonders of a good sleep.

This story shows how important sleep is in our lives, and how we often take it for granted until things get out of hand like they did for the GBI agent. As I mentioned in the Introduction, sleep affects how we work, relate to other people, make decisions, as well as how we *feel*. The idea that we need to "sleep on it" when faced with a big decision is no joke. We intuitively know that sleep helps us think better, stronger, and prepares our minds for optimal functionality. (And, in case you don't believe me, a Dutch study released in 2006 and published in the journal *Science* points to the benefits of taking in information and letting the "unconscious" mind during sleep churn through the options involved in making complex decisions. Other experiments have also backed this finding, proving that sleep helps the brain commit new information to memory by way of a process called memory consolidation.)

This all bodes well for those who can enjoy perfect sleep night after night. But getting a good night's sleep is hard for many.

Sleep as a topic has gotten a lot of attention recently—and for good reason. The science is finally catching up to and confirming all the anecdotal evidence that's been mounting. As I indicated in the Introduction, inadequate sleep translates to poorer health, obesity, lower productivity on the job—including the job of being a full-time parent— more danger on the roads, a less vibrant sex life, and a lower quality of life. In fact, researchers have found that after two weeks, people sleeping four to six hours a night are as cognitively impaired as those who have been awake for two or three days.

Combined with new research are the results of polls taken on Americans that demonstrate the extent of our sleep problems. Not only does routine sleep loss takes its toll, but routine sleep loss is also a routine occurrence in America. The majority of us frequently have a symptom of a sleep problem, including frequent waking during the night or snoring. These problems are bad enough that a quarter of us admit that our daily activities are affected. A quarter of us with partners say our sexual relationships have suffered from lack of sleep, and that we've been having less sex or have lost interest in sex entirely. Sixty percent of us have driven while drowsy in the past year, and some of us (about 4 percent) have had an accident or a close call because we were too tired or fell asleep at the wheel. One study released in April 2006 reported that drowsiness contributed to 20 percent of all crashes and 16 percent of near crashes in a year-long examination of 241 drivers in the Washington, D.C., area.

And, let's be honest: We look like a sleep-deprived society.

The problem is serious, and given the fact that our doctors are not likely to ask us about our sleep, it's easy to avoid recognizing and dealing with the problem.

> An estimated 20 million people have sleep apnea, a common medical disorder that disrupts sleep night after night, causing daytime sleepiness and, in some cases, weight gain. Millions of these adults and children have no idea they have this problem, which is easily treatable. See "Diagnosing a Sleep Disorder" on page 30 to see if you're potentially one of these sufferers. Sleep apnea is more than just a sleep problem; it is associated with hypertension, stroke, automobile accidents, mood and memory problems, and heart disease.

I can tell you from a personal standpoint that sleep is essential. I know I need it and I know I must have it to function. But, like everyone else, when my stress level is high and I take a lot of anxieties to bed, sleep doesn't come as easily.

I know that without sleep, several physiological things will happen: My reaction time will slow down; my mental-processing time will slow down; I can make poor decisions; I'll be irritable, moody, and low in stamina. Lack of sleep or too much sleep also can be signs of illness (lack of sleep is associated with over forty different medical causes, and excess sleep can be a sign of a sleep disorder or depression). If I go without quality sleep my immune function will suffer, and I might gain weight more easily. I know that sleep is a basic drive or function of which the scientific cause is still unknown. There are several theories, but none are definitive. Even though my career is about teaching good sleep habits and changing other people's lives through sleep, I still have my own personal struggles with juggling a demanding work and family life with achieving quality sleep every single night no matter what. I do, however, prioritize sleep. And I consider myself to be a relatively good sleeper.

Sleep is the ultimate research topic. Although we have a better understanding of sleep today than we did twenty years ago, research is still in its germinal stages. We don't even know why we sleep. It seems to be such a basic question that deserves a clear answer, but there is none—yet. The amount of sleep you get—and its quality—is more important than previously thought. We've known for some time that lack of sleep causes foggy thinking and poor concentration, but now we also know that chronic lack of sleep can put you at risk for type 2 diabetes and obesity. Lack of sleep also impairs your immune system, putting you at risk for colds and other infections. We know that REM—rapid eye movement—sleep affects memory, that some people need more (or less) sleep than others, that there are genetic expressions for sleepiness, and that there is a distinct physiological process that occurs when the body sleeps, or *doesn't*. We know what disrupts sleep (or at least we think we do), but we don't have a great number of effective ways to treat these disruptions. Finally, we know that sleep deprivation is torturous. Terrorists and intelligence agents alike will starve an individual of sleep as a form of torture and in an attempt to pry out information. It was a tactic favored by the KGB and the Japanese in prisoner-of-war camps during World War II. Sleep deprivation may even be one of the oldest forms of torture, a way to induce paranoia, disorientation, and even hallucinations without any drugs. The ancient Romans referred to sleep deprivation as *tormentum vigilae*, or "waking torture," which they used to extract information from their enemies.

We are just starting to get an understanding of what sleep disorders are out there, and are still trying to discover how to treat them. We have little idea of how to treat *disordered* sleep, or even what that truly means. (I'll define the difference between a sleep disorder and disordered sleep shortly.)

The topics related to sleep are endless, which presents its own problems. What do we study first? The roots of a sleeping disorder? Or why does getting quality sleep keep our waistlines in check? It's a challenge to wrap your brain around it all. This is a mountainous subject and we're standing at the bottom with our climbing gear on. Not much got accomplished in the realm of sleep science between 350 B.C., when Aristotle wrote, "A person awakes from sleep when digestion is completed," and 1900, when Sigmund Freud's *The Interpretation of Dreams* was published.

> Dr. Nathaniel Kleitman is universally recognized as "the father of American sleep research." One of his students, Dr. William Dement, went on to also become a pioneering sleep researcher, describing the cyclical nature of sleep and establishing the relationship between REM sleep and dreaming. Whether or not Dr. Kleitman can credit good sleep habits to his longevity is anyone's guess; born before Freud published his seminal work, Dr. Kleitman lived to be 104 years old and died in 1999. Dr. Dement continues on as an advocate for funding of sleep research and to teach the value of sleep to all who will listen.

Unlike other fields of medicine, very little sleep research was done prior to 1953, when Dr. Nathaniel Kleitman and Dr. Eugene Aserinsky discovered rapid eye movement (REM) at the University of Chicago. Although sleep research gained momentum in the second half of the twentieth century, led by people like Dr. William C. Dement, who founded the first sleep center at Stanford University in 1970 (this was preceded by the first narcolepsy clinic in Walla Walla, Washington), it wasn't until 1990 that the National Sleep Foundation was founded to improve public health and safety through a better understanding of sleep and sleep disorders. This was the year *after* the *Exxon Valdez* tanker ran aground on Bligh Reef, in Prince William Sound, Alaska, when its driver allegedly succumbed to fatigue in the wheelhouse and caused one of the largest oil spills in history. That event clearly demonstrated the toll that sleep deprivation can take on all of us indirectly through other people. When you consider how much of your life depends on others making good decisions—doctors, industrial workers, pilots, air-traffic controllers, drivers, train conductors, presidents, world leaders, and so on—you soon realize that sleep deprivation isn't just about you. It's about everyone.

> Sleep debt increases your chances of falling asleep when you least expect it, including taking "microsleeps," which are seconds-long daytime dips into sleep that happen when sleep-type brain-wave activity crosses over those waking brain waves. Such microsleeps can result in slips and falls, or in more serious mistakes that threaten public safety. The National Highway Traffic Safety Administration estimates that each year, drowsiness causes 100,000 vehicle crashes, resulting in 76,000 injuries and 1,500 deaths.

The point of this book is not to exhume the scientific and philosophical reasoning behind sleep. That won't help you attain better sleeping skills or peel five years off your face. I want to teach you how to sleep better so you can get the most out of life, feel good, and look younger. It's possible, and you'd be surprised by how easy it can be to make little changes to your sleeping habits that translate to big health rewards.

> No one really knows why we sleep. There are several theories out there, including restoration of bodily function, memory consolidation, and energy conservation, all of which have been proven and disproven with current research.

Before we undertake the hands-on process of working toward achieving great sleep, I want you to understand a few concepts, which will provide the foundation you need for familiarizing yourself with your current sleep habits, identifying your troubled areas, and improving your sleep. The following is a list of vocabulary words I'll use throughout the book:

- sleep debt
- quality versus quantity of sleep
- sleep disorders versus disordered sleep
- diagnosing a sleep disorder

- insomnia symptoms or syndrome
- sleep hygiene

SLEEP DEPRIVATION = SLEEP DEBT

It's true that we sleep less today than ever before. In fact, in just the past 100 years alone, Americans have cut their sleep time by about 20 percent. How we sleep has had a few major changes over the centuries based on some interesting historical developments. The introduction of the lightbulb in 1879 suddenly changed how long people could work. We then had the possibility of a twenty-four-hour society, and sleep habits had to change for those working the third shift. Another big issue was the proliferation of caffeine in consumable drinks as an alerting agent, which prevents sleep or at least replaces it for a short while. The concept of overtime has also changed sleep habits, encouraging many to utilize overtime for more money. In a perfect world, you'd earn *less* for working more, thus encouraging good sleep habits so there is no financial incentive to miss out on sleep.

Our lifestyles leave little time for sleep, and our society motivates people to work and play more, and sleep less. Economic necessity plus family demands often compel us to throw sleep out the window without even thinking about it. We worry about everything else in our lives before we worry about sleep. And our priorities reflect this inevitable reality. You know from your own experience that stress can morph into psychological problems like anxiety, nervousness, depression . . . and ultimately lost sleep. But sometimes it's hard to admit that our psychological issues are having a deep impact on our ability to sleep.

> For many, sleep is not a priority. It gets in the way of doing other things. There are strong financial incentives to sleep less. We don't count how many dreams we have in the bank; we count dollars.

So what's your sleep debt? The answer to that question comes with knowing exactly how many hours you need each and every night. Not everyone is created equal in this equation. I need seven hours of sleep a night to feel refreshed and alert all day long, whereas you might need nine hours, or only 6.5. Your sleep needs might also vary depending on what's going on in your life. You may need more sleep during times of acute stress, grief, hard work, physical training, illness, or depression. Your sleep habits might also change with age, which we'll explore shortly. In general, if you need only five hours or less, you're considered a short sleeper; if you need ten hours or more, you're said to be a long sleeper. (To distinguish, "light" sleeper refers to people who are easily awakened and may not experience as much deep sleep. Short sleepers, on the other hand, can have lots of deep sleep but not need as many hours of sleep. So "light" refers to quality or type of sleep whereas "short" refers to duration of sleep—five hours or less.)

Is there such thing as sleeping too much? If you sleep more than nine hours a night, for instance, should you aim to cut *back* on your sleep time? This very question has only recently sparked scientific testing. Because insomniacs and sleep-deprived people often get the attention, few wonder what the potential health risks are for those who sleep long nights—more than nine hours. Some studies have documented the health risks of long sleepers. For example, one study found that long sleepers had a 50 percent greater risk of stroke than did those who slept six to eight hours a night. They may also have higher rates of cardiovascular disease, depression, and possibly an increased risk for diabetes. A large Japanese study found that those who slept more than 7.5 hours had a greater mortality risk than those who slept less than 6.5 hours. But don't let this alarm you. These studies cannot make any definitive conclusions yet because the explanations behind their results aren't clear, and there are just as many other studies to complicate some of this new evidence. For example, research suggests that women who are, in fact, longer sleepers may have a lower risk of breast cancer. Confusing?

Obviously, distinguishing between fact and fiction is still up for debate. Suffice it to say there is no magical number for sleep that covers everybody's needs. Sleep needs vary with each individual. If you're a long sleeper who feels lethargic much of the day—which many people experience after spending too much time in bed on weekends and vacations—you just might benefit from restricting your time in bed. (Regulating your sleep schedule using my programs will help you do this.) The point is to find which number of hours makes you feel the best, and then aim to sleep that number every night. Whether it's seven hours or nine doesn't matter.

In Chapter 8 I'll take you through an exercise that will help you determine your number—your individual sleep need in hours. Thus, if you know you need eight hours a night and you only get seven hours for eight straight days, then you have lost one full night's sleep (eight hours) after those eight days. You probably know if you're chronically sleep deprived without having to take a test. It's not rocket science. Much like being thirsty, your body tells you when you're missing something it wants.

Focus less on calculating your total sleep debt and, instead, concentrate on moving forward with practicing better sleep habits. Your body will respond and deposit lost sleep back into its "bank" naturally.

> Sleep deprivation is cumulative, building a sleep debt that must be paid. Losing as little as one and a half hours for just one night reduces daytime alertness by about one-third. Excessive daytime sleepiness impairs memory and the ability to think and process information. Sleep deprivation also leads to mood alterations, attention deficits, slower reaction times, and an increased risk for accidents.

> **Q.** Is a sleep debt reversible? Can I pay back a sleep debt?
> **A.** Yes, you can catch up on sleep and refill that sleep bank over time with quality, restful sleep.
> **Q.** Can I bank sleep for later?
> **A.** No, unfortunately it doesn't seem to work that way. But if you know you're going to have a night that requires you to forgo some sleep time for a special situation, then a well-planned nap may be the answer (see Chapter 7).

Gender, Age, and Sleep

I get asked all the time if a woman or a man needs more sleep. This is a hard question to answer because the research just isn't there yet. Beyond what the scientific reports tell me, what I see in actual people day in and day out from a clinical perspective, however, says a lot. I know from a clinical standpoint that women tend to confess more about sleep issues than men. Does that mean men are less vulnerable to sleep problems or that women happen to be more comfortable talking about their health? It's hard to say. Given my experience I'm inclined to admit that women, as a gender, appear to bear numerous stresses due to the multifaceted nature of their roles in today's society: Mom. Wife. Employee. Chauffeur. Cook. Cleaner. Business owner. Family manager. Caretaker, etc. When I sit and talk with my female patients—who do happen to comprise more of my patient base than males—we discuss everything from pregnancy to menopause, to career, to marriage, and that word "balance," and I know I've got it much easier than many of them.

One would naturally think that since women and men are physiologically different, they'd also have different sleep needs. But women, from adolescence to postmenopause, are underrepresented in studies of sleep and its disorders. Although sleep complaints are twice as prevalent among women, the majority of sleep research has been conducted in men (this is changing). Some studies are now showing that women may be at greater risk for insomnia, or have a predisposition due to their sex, but explaining this from a purely scientific standpoint is not entirely possible right now. Thus, the question remains unanswered.

Compounding the complexity of this question is the fact that age can have more to do with sleep needs and experiences than gender. For example, younger women may build up a sleep debt more easily than older women. Whether or not this is true, however, is debatable. In fact, many sleep studies result in controversial and inconclusive data.

> Q. Does the amount of sleep we need really decrease as we age, or is that hearsay?
>
> A. The amount of sleep we need remains constant, but this has been debated. The older we get, the harder it becomes to meet our sleep needs, for a variety of reasons. Even if we're able to function better with less sleep the older we get, that doesn't mean our bodies don't, in fact, crave that sleep. Older people take more daytime naps to make up for poor sleep at night, which can be due to medicinal or medical causes, or simply having more time to sleep.

What we do know about sleep and aging is that the older you get, the more likely you are to suffer from interrupted sleep, which is critical to feeling rested and refreshed. Older people still need roughly the same number of sleep hours as they got when they were younger (it may deviate by thirty minutes to an hour, over a lifetime), but the architecture of their sleep shifts. The amplitude (height) of their brain waves decreases, making these waves no longer meet criteria for deep sleep. They are easily awakened by noise, light, or even their own pain from a chronic medical condition. Sleep becomes more fragmented and inefficient, so the actual time spent sleeping is less than the time spent in bed.

Another influential aspect of aging that can affect sleep is your circadian rhythm, which is a very important subject matter we'll be visiting throughout this book. Circadian rhythms are the patterns of repeated activity associated with the environmental cycles of day and night. Our internal rhythms repeat roughly every twenty-four hours. Examples include the sleep-wake cycle, the ebb and flow of hormones, the rise and fall of body temperature, and other subtle rhythms that mesh with the twenty-four-hour solar day. A lot of people's sleep problems can be attributed to an internal clock that has become out of sync or mismatched with the day-night cycle. And as you'll learn about extensively, light has an immense impact on setting our body clocks, also called our circadian pacemakers.

Everyone's circadian pacemaker ticks at a different rate, but as you age, your pacemaker will speed up or slow down, thus altering how your body responds to that twenty-four-hour cycle. Babies don't get a rhythm going until about six months of age, at which point they establish a rhythm that matches closely with the twenty-four-hour day. If you've had teenagers in the house, you know they typically don't go to bed much before eleven at night. From the age of about fifteen to twenty-five, that pacemaker slows down, so a seventeen-year-old's body usually won't want to go to sleep early or get up early. Sometime during our late twenties, the body clock speeds back up again so it matches the twenty-four-hour day. Then, later on in life, our clocks speed up further, so the body doesn't match so well with the twenty-four-hour day. It wants to go to bed early and get up super early, which is what you find Granny and Gramps doing. At an older age the body also doesn't experience as strong a fluctuation in core body temperature throughout the day, which affects the rhythm. This might explain partially why older people's rhythms aren't as robust and clearly defined as younger people's. Older people will weave in and out of being semi-sleepy and semi-awake throughout the day and night.

Science is still trying to understand completely how our body clocks work, and even how *many* body clocks we have. Currently, we think we have two body clocks: one that is set by outward cues of light and darkness, and a second one that has an internal schedule set in the brain. It is when these two clocks don't agree on the same schedule, and compete with each other, that we feel "off." Synchronizing these two clocks comes with hitting the "reset" button every twenty-four hours. We can do this by exposure to light and by activity. For example, when you want to be alert and awake but your body doesn't want to follow, you can stimulate your body to reset itself just by going outside into the sunlight for ten or fifteen minutes or engaging in some physical activity, preferably outside in the bright light. (Much more on this topic later on.)

QUALITY AND QUANTITY

If you wake up after seven to eight hours of sleep and still feel unrefreshed, your problem may not be about quantity but rather *quality*. The quality of sleep is as vitally important to our health and well-being as is the quantity. Why? Our sleep has a complex pattern, or architecture, that cycles through five stages during the night. During certain stages and times of the sleep cycles, we secrete hormones and other substances that help regulate our metabolism and support our general health. As you'll learn about in Chapter 5, the secretion of growth hormone during deep sleep is important for repairing and replenishing cells. What happens in our brains during REM sleep is how we retain information, organize our memories, and prepare to learn something new or perform a special task. If our sleep patterns are altered, it may leave us feeling unrefreshed, tired, and sleepy, as well as put us at risk for a host of minor and even serious medical conditions.

Q. Can I get physically sick from lack of sleep? If I pull an all-nighter and then catch a cold, can I blame the sleepless night for the cold?

A. Immunologists and sleep researchers have tried to put this one to the test. Anecdotal evidence from people's personal experiences suggests a link between sleep and susceptibility to illness. Studies do suggest that the quality of your sleep prior to infection factors into whether you catch a cold and, if so, how severe it is. Some studies even suggest that those who get six hours or less of sleep have 50 percent less immunity protection than those who get eight hours per night. Certain cells that modulate the immune system increase during sleep, so missing out on sleep means your resistance to viral infection drops. And, in fact, researchers have found that when recipients are sleep deprived, the flu shot is less effective.

If sleep weren't so key to immune health, then we'd probably not experience that compelling need to sleep when we're coming down with an illness.

SLEEP DISORDER VERSUS DISORDERED SLEEP

Wake up to this simple fact: You are not supposed to be sleepy, with your feet dragging and lids lagging during the day. If you are asleep literally before your head hits the pillow, this may not be a good sign. Do not let the notion "I have always been this way" fool you into thinking it's okay. You should awaken feeling relatively refreshed and remain alert throughout the day—every day.

If you don't, it could be the result of one of two problems: a sleep disorder, or simply disordered sleep. What's the difference?

The distinction between a sleep disorder and what I call "disordered sleep" is important. Think of sleep disorders as formal syndromes with definitive criteria, which repeat time after time. They can be primary sleep disorders, which are not attributed to other conditions; or secondary sleep disorders that arise from an underlying physical or mental condition. For example, restless legs syndrome (RLS) is a type of sleep disorder. Insomnia, while it can be defined as a formal sleep disorder, has variants that, on the other hand, may be due to depression or some other underlying physiological cause that warrants treatment. Often, a primary sleep disorder can give rise to a secondary sleep disorder. For example, someone who has restless legs syndrome also may develop insomnia as a result of his or her chronic inability to sleep soundly. This is when treating the symptoms of the primary sleep disorder often improves symptoms of other sleep disorders.

The criteria that define disorders are developed and agreed upon by national researchers and societies to help the medical field understand how to identify a particular set of circumstances. And once a disorder has been identified, the goal is to systematically develop a therapy to treat the symptoms associated with it, or cure the underlying situation. There are more than eighty-five recognized sleep disorders, the most recognizable of which may be insomnia, sleep apnea, narcolepsy, and restless legs syndrome. These and others may manifest themselves in various ways.

> The most common type of disordered sleep I see in my practice is non-refreshing sleep. A patient will come in and say she's been waking up after enough sleep but feels like she's slept poorly. This can be caused by several things:
>
> - poor diet
> - stress
> - environment
> - genetics
>
> My goal is then to figure out which of these—if not a combination of them—is the culprit, and find an action or actions to take. The most common treatments I give to help someone sleep better include the following:
>
> - behavioral techniques
> - relaxation techniques
> - environmental tips
> - suggestions for medications or supplements to discuss with their physician
>
> By the end of this book, you'll have learned about all of these tricks.

"Disordered sleep" refers to everything else that relates to sleep but does not qualify as a disorder. One's symptoms might not quite meet the disorder criteria based on severity or frequency, or there might be an external behavioral factor that's affecting sleep, such as a cat in the bed or too much heat in the room. Disordered sleep can also reflect the value we place (or don't place) on sleep, or the quality of sleep we get.

For the vast majority of people, disordered sleep is the biggest culprit. In fact, sleep problems often occur as the result of poor "sleep hygiene"—bad habits that don't support a good sleep experience. Such habits entail a range of practices and environmental factors, many of which are under your control. They include things like smoking, drinking alcohol or caffeine, vigorous exercise or eating a large meal before bed, jet lag from travel across time zones, and psychological stressors like deadlines, exams, marital conflict, and job crises that intrude on your ability to fall asleep or stay asleep. Designing and sticking with a good sleep hygiene program, which you're going to do in the programs outlined, should alleviate these types of problems, or at least give you a disciplined way to handle them so that they minimally affect your sleep.

DIAGNOSING A SLEEP DISORDER

The idea that sleep disorders can be life-threatening when they go undiagnosed is an old finding but one we could only recently prove. The research keeps accumulating on how much sleep disorders can influence or exacerbate serious health conditions. Obstructive sleep apnea, for example, which causes sleeping people to temporarily stop breathing, more than doubles the chances of a stroke or death. Particularly severe cases of this disorder can more than triple the risk of stroke or death. The prevalence of sleep apnea is on par with that of diabetes and asthma combined. Twenty-four percent of adult men and 9 percent of adult women—or more than 20 million Americans—are estimated to have some degree of obstructive sleep apnea. Only a fraction of these have been diagnosed and treated by a physician.

About one-third of the 5 million Americans with heart failure also have central sleep apnea. Central sleep apnea is different from obstructive; in central, your brain tells your lungs not to breathe, whereas in obstructive, your lungs work but your throat's muscles relax and close your airway partially or completely.

Symptoms of sleep disorders can occur when trying to sleep, during sleep, and while awake at various times during the day. Sleep disorders are tricky; individual symptoms may be present in one or more sleep disorders, as well as in conditions unrelated to sleep problems. If you do have a sleep disorder, you need to visit a sleep specialist who can diagnose exactly your medical problem and treat it accordingly (see Appendix B for resources). Nonetheless, this book can help you rule out the possibility that modifying your sleep habits can help relieve your problems. If you already know you've got a sleep disorder, or receive such a diagnosis in the future, use this book to create the best environment for sleep, which will help you manage your sleep disorder and increase the chances that you'll routinely experience a good night's sleep.

To get a sense of where you stand, ask yourself the following questions. Have you ever regularly:

- awakened after seven to eight hours of sleep feeling un-refreshed?
- spontaneously fallen asleep during meetings or social events?
- gotten a creepy, crawly sensation in your legs, with an irresistible urge to move them, especially when you lie down in bed at night?
- found that your bed partner has vanished sometime in the night because your snoring was not a melodic symphony, or that you literally kicked your partner out of bed?

If any of this rings true, you may have a sleep problem, a medical sleep disorder, or a related medical condition for which treatment may literally change your life. Obviously, awakening after a night's sleep still feeling un-refreshed may be explained easily with a look at the habits and behaviors under your control. But it can also point to a real medical disorder. Many sleep disorders are secondary to a variety of medical and mental-health disorders, pain, and even the treatments for these disorders. Medical conditions like diabetes, congestive heart failure, emphysema, stroke, and others may have nighttime symptoms that disturb sleep. Depressive illnesses and anxiety disorders are also associated with sleep disturbances, as is the pain from conditions like arthritis, cancer, and acid reflux.

Recognizing and distinguishing among sleep problems, primary sleep disorders, and those secondary to or associated with medical conditions is essential to proper diagnosis and treatment. It is equally important, however, to realize that they often interact in a complex manner, with each impacting the other. For example, poor sleep can affect your mood, and your mood can affect the quality of your sleep. Poor sleep can contribute to obesity, and obesity can cause sleep disorders. Exactly how all these factors interact is not completely known, but we can target each aspect individually to achieve vastly improved interventions and treatments.

I suggest that you use this book to attain better sleep habits, and if you're still not getting the results you need, consider seeing a specialist.

The magnitude of the impact of sleep disorders on our individual and public health, safety, and performance is truly enormous. Fortunately, increasing awareness is leading to more effective treatment, less suffering, and happier, more productive lives.

The Most Common Sleep Disorders

Apnea. Your patient and empathic bed partner notices that you suddenly cease not only your snoring, but your breathing as well. You actually stop breathing, for ten, then twenty, then thirty seconds. Then, to his or her surprise, you begin to gasp for air as if it were your last breath. This cycle repeats itself over and over, all night long. For your part, you may be totally unaware of all of that, as the alarm clock rings. You may wake up with a dry mouth, a headache, and feeling hungover. You may also be sleepy during the day; have significant memory loss; have concentration, attention, mood, and other related problems. This rather horrifying scenario is typical for a disorder called sleep apnea. With obstructive sleep apnea, the lungs continue to work but the muscles in the throat become so relaxed that the airway becomes all or partially closed. With central sleep apnea, a far rarer form, the body temporarily stops making any effort to breathe.

Potential signs of sleep apnea that can go under the radar are the following:

- getting up during the night to urinate (Reason: Light sleep caused by apnea will have a lower wake threshold and cause you to wake up more easily in response to the urge to urinate. That need to urinate happens because apnea can stress the heart, which leads muscle cells to release a substance that then triggers the kidneys to produce urine.)
- decreased interest in sex; or impotence (Reason: Sleep deprivation caused by the apnea may lead to impotence; however, studies showing the link between apnea and erectile dysfunction are not entirely conclusive.)
- needing two or more medicines to control blood pressure (Reason: Unknown, but statistics show a relationship between difficult-to-manage hypertension and obstructive sleep apnea.)
- heartburn during sleep (Reason: Generally speaking, patients with sleep apnea often complain of heartburn during sleep. It's unclear, however, which comes first—the heartburn or the apnea. It may be a vicious cycle since both cause inflammation in the airway, which leads to reflux and sleep apnea.)
- falling asleep at the movies or watching TV (Reason: Apnea causes fragmented sleep, which then translates to daytime sleepiness.)

Bruxism. A more common problem than most people think, bruxism occurs when you wake up with a tension headache or a sore jaw from grinding or clenching your teeth while you sleep. Dentists are usually good with monitoring your teeth and looking for signs of damage. Treatments range from mouth guards to meditation.

Restless legs syndrome (RLS). Particularly around bedtime, many people (about 10 to 15 percent of the population) experience "pins and needles feelings," an "internal itch," or a "creeping, crawling sensation" in their legs, with a subsequent irresistible urge to relieve this discomfort by vigorously moving their legs. RLS makes it difficult to fall asleep, and a related disorder—periodic limb movements—may also awaken you out of sleep, forcing you to walk around to relieve the discomfort. Symptoms of RLS can range from being bothersome to having a severe impact on your and your bed partner's lives. The exact cause of RLS is unknown, and it is considered a neurologic sensorimotor disorder. Primary RLS accounts for 40 to 60 percent of all cases and is not related to other disorders. Secondary RLS is a form related to an underlying condition such as kidney failure, pregnancy, or iron deficiency anemia. Certain medications can trigger or worsen this form. Lots of research is currently under way to understand and treat RLS.

Narcolepsy. Excessive daytime sleepiness is typically the first symptom. It's the overwhelming need to sleep when you prefer to be awake. Narcolepsy is associated with a sudden weakness or paralysis often initiated by laughter or other intense feelings; sleep paralysis, an often frightening situation, where one is half awake yet cannot move; and intensely vivid and scary dreams occurring at the onset or end of sleep. One may also experience automatic behavior, in which one performs routine or boring tasks without full memory later.

Periodic limb movements. These can be anything from small twitches to full kicks that occur within ninety seconds of each other throughout the night. You may not realize that these movements can wake you up, but you do wake to an unrefreshed feeling in the morning.

Insomnia. This is the inability to fall asleep or stay asleep, or waking too early, for more than four to five nights per week, and for more than two to three months (see below for more details).

If you suspect you have a sleep disorder, this book is a starting point for ruling out other potential problems that you can control on your own. If, after you've gone through my programs, you still cannot get a good night's sleep, speak to your primary care physician and consider seeing a sleep specialist. Combined with the guidance of your doctor and/or a sleep specialist, this book remains a good source of information for working through your sleep issues.

INSOMNIACS ON THE RISE

When we think about sleep disorders, insomnia quickly comes to mind. We immediately recall the last time we couldn't fall asleep easily, or when we woke up at 3 A.M. only to stare at the alarm clock until 4 A.M. knowing it would go off in a few short hours. Insomnia is like a demon who enters our minds at night when we're supposed to be blissfully asleep, preventing us from getting the Zs our bodies long for. This demon is hard to tame, hard to evict from our bedrooms when we've got so much to think and worry about.

Where Do You Fit In?

The following is a summary of some of the results from a 2005 "Sleep in America" poll conducted by the National Sleep Foundation. How do you measure up?

- On average, adults are sleeping 6.8 hours a night on weekdays and 7.4 hours a night on weekends. Overall, adults report sleeping an average of 6.9 hours a night when considering both weekday and weekend sleep.
- Twenty-six percent of adults say they have "a good night's sleep" only a few nights a month or less.
- On average, people say they need a minimum of 6.5 hours of sleep a night to function at their best during the day. In general, men report needing less sleep (6.2 hours) than women (6.8 hours) to function at their best.
- When asked if they feel they are more alert, productive, and energetic in the morning or in the evening, more than one-half (55 percent) report that they are morning people (larks), while 41 percent consider themselves evening people (owls).
- More than one-half (55 percent) take, on average, at least one nap during the week, with one-third (35 percent) reporting that they take two or more naps.
- About one-half (47 percent) report that, on weeknights, they stay up later than they planned or wanted to at least a few nights a week. Three in ten adults (30 percent) say that they rarely or never stay up later than anticipated. Those who stay up later than they planned at least a few nights a week are about twice as likely than those who rarely or never do so to be on the Internet (34 percent versus 19 percent) and/or doing work related to their job (23 percent versus 11 percent).
- On average, it takes about twenty-three minutes to fall asleep on most nights.

In 2006, the foundation focused on teens and found that America's youth aren't getting the sleep they need, either. Interestingly, parents think their kids are getting enough sleep, but the kids know they're not! Caffeine and tech toys are as much sleep thieves for teens as they are for adults. The study also found that parents play a key role in helping their adolescent children get a good night's sleep. This, in turn, affects their moods, education, and driving abilities. For more on this poll, go to www.sleepfoundation.org.

Insomnia affects more than 70 million Americans, or one in three people; more than half of adults encounter this demon a few nights a week or more. Direct costs of insomnia, which include dollars spent on insomnia treatment, health care services, hospital and nursing home care, are estimated at nearly $14 billion annually. Indirect costs such as work loss, property damage from accidents, and transportation to and from health care providers are estimated to be $28 billion. Although insomnia is the most common sleep problem among roughly one-half of older adults, they are less likely to experience frequent symptoms of insomnia than their younger counterparts (45 percent versus 62 percent), and their symptoms are more likely to be associated with medical conditions.

But is insomnia (which literally means "no sleep," or the inability to sleep) a real disorder in itself or just a symptom of, say, stress and anxiety? For a long time, doctors were told insomnia was merely a symptom of other conditions, but new evidence is beginning to suggest it may be a disorder in its own right. Regardless of whether it occurs with other medical conditions or by itself, insomnia tends to have a consistent set of nighttime and daytime symptoms. The three characteristics of insomnia include difficulty going to sleep, difficulty staying asleep, and waking too early in the morning. This results in inadequate or poor quality sleep, which carries with it a host of potential consequences. For starters, insomnia is a risk factor for the onset of depression and can significantly affect your quality of life. Not getting enough good sleep can result in daytime fatigue, impaired mood, depression and psychological distress, and decreased ability to concentrate, problem-solve, and make decisions, as well as being at risk for injury, driving drowsy, and illness.

If you're among the millions who do suffer from insomnia, whether chronically or occasionally, this book can help you target some of the possible underlying problems and guide you through techniques to tame them. It can also be used in conjunction with formal treatment given by a sleep specialist.

THE ROBBERS OF A GOOD NIGHT'S REST

Sleep needs and patterns may be unique to each individual, but the typical thieves of restful sleep are not. In my practice, I hear time and time again the same complaints and discover that the roots of the problems—of disordered sleep—typically fall under one of six categories:

- anxiety, stress, and nervousness
- caffeine consumption
- parenting
- bed partners
- hormonal fluctuations (culprits of either the X or Y chromosome)
- traveling, especially business traveling

Maybe you have issues under more than one of these categories. For example, you may be a working mother who uses caffeine to stay alert through the day, struggles to juggle work and home life, has a husband whose sleep habits don't jibe with your own, and experiences severe hormonal fluctuations through the month that impact your sleep-wake cycle. Sound familiar?

In Chapters 2 and 3 I'm going to take you through evaluating and dealing with each of these sleep thieves. You'll get a quick 101 education on each culprit as well as the lessons you need to make shifts in your lifestyle today and see immediate results. I'm always surprised to hear that most people would not speak with their doctor if they thought they had a sleep problem. Many assume the problem would go away. Maybe it will go away.

But chances are, it won't.

If you only get the average of 6.8 hours of sleep a night on weekdays and 7.4 hours a night on weekends, but you could really use a full eight hours every night, you're racking up almost fifty nights of lost sleep in one year! A debt that must be paid.

SLEEP HYGIENE

Like other sleep doctors, I call the practices, habits, and environmental factors in your life that are critically important for sound sleep your "sleep hygiene," a concept I've already touched upon and will revisit throughout the book. Good sleep hygiene can have a tremendous impact on getting better sleep. With this book, you'll be able to develop your own sleep hygiene practices that fit your individual needs. Just as not everyone's sleep requirements will be the same, not everyone's sleep hygiene practices will be identical, either. You will also have to consider special circumstances that you alone might have, such as a serious case of insomnia, troubled sleep related to pregnancy, or signs of a sleep disorder.

The way our society runs today makes it a challenge to prioritize sleep, and we fight our needs to sleep every day. We have twenty-four-hour supermarkets and pharmacies, cable TV with round-the-clock coverage, and an Internet full of information, entertainment, and communication that never gets turned off. Include your daily responsibilities and activities, and you've got a potential To Do list that occupies every hour of the day—and night. The mere thought of living a twenty-four-hour life is tiring, isn't it?

Sleep Around the World

- Seventy-five percent of people in Portugal stay up past midnight, the highest percentage of any country.
- Seven of the top ten nocturnal areas are in Asia, led by Taiwan, where 69 percent turn in after midnight.
- The Japanese sleep less than anyone else on the planet, with 41 percent snoozing just six hours or less each night.
- Australians go to bed the earliest and sleep the longest. In a poll, nearly one-quarter of Australians said they go bed by 10 P.M., and 31 percent said they average more than nine hours of sleep every night.

Fully half of us are often tired, fatigued, or just don't feel up to our usual energy during the day, and 17 percent say they feel this way almost every day. Half of us get a good night's sleep nearly every night, but the other half sleeps well only a few nights a month or less. What I find most stunning is the fact that few of these poor sleepers believe they have a problem, or they choose to ignore it.

Despite the hormones and genetics that have a lot of control over you and your appearance, by understanding which factors in your life *you* can control, you can ultimately be the decision maker when it comes to determining how fast you age. In other words, I want *you* to hold that remote control. It's possible, and I'll show you exactly how. Then the transformation will begin. Remember: Getting quality sleep is the new vital sign of health.

CHAPTER 2

The Three Most Troublesome Culprits in Disordered Sleep . . . and How to Conquer Them

When was the last time you went through your day feeling exceptionally alert and refreshed? Was it yesterday? The day before that?

You're not alone if you can't come up with that day easily. Today more adults are experiencing sleep problems on a regular basis than they were ten years ago. Most of us are walking around with some level of sleepiness. And if I were to ask what's your excuse for not getting your Zs, you'd probably blame your list of To Dos, work, stress, kids, a restless bed partner, or physical reasons. These, alongside a few tangential factors, are among the most common culprits in disordered sleep. In fact, through my work and clinical experience I've found six distinct reasons persist for poor-quality sleep—all of which may be alleviated by simple lifestyle modifications. I've categorized these six culprits into two groups: 1) those that arise from specific biological effects that are more or less "invisible" to you because you feel them from within you— namely, the effects of caffeine, anxiety, and your gender; and 2) those that arise from a broader range of effects that result from your role as a parent, a frequent traveler, or a bed partner.

Starting in this chapter and extending into Chapter 3, you're going to find out which of these six sleep thieves impact you the most, and how you can start fixing the problem today. You may already have a good idea of what disturbs your sleep. Then again, you may not. So be sure to take all of the quizzes. Your responses might surprise you.

Kathy's Story

Kathy W. was told she was going to have to move across the country due to her husband's new job. She was a stay-at-home mother of three and had a history of mild to moderate depression. She also ran her own small business as a calligrapher and stationery designer from home. Kathy prepared herself for the move as best she could, but several stressful events happened beyond her control. First, the move itself was difficult—getting the family packed, organizing and managing the trucks and movers, prepping and selling the house, as well as purchasing a new one (timed perfectly, no less). Stress took on a whole new meaning for Kathy. Her small business had been a great source of personal fulfillment and stress relief, but she had to close up shop indefinitely until she was reestablished in her new home. She handled the transition well at the start with the support of a solid network of friends and her husband's help.

The closer the day got to the actual move, the harder it became for Kathy to get quality sleep, as she found herself going over lists in her head, staying up at night (she was a bit of a night owl, anyway), flipping TV channels, and drinking more coffee during the mornings. When she, the kids, pets, and her husband finally made the trip across the country, it was hard on her. The moving truck was late, and they had to stay in a hotel for a week before the new house was ready—all while her husband was trying to begin a new job. As the stress piled up, Kathy experienced more restless nights. One night she tried to practice her calligraphy as a way to relax, but it gave her more anxiety about not having worked in several weeks. She managed to get the kids into a new routine at their new school, but she couldn't get her business going again quickly because the house needed lots of work, and settling into a different environment and location proved a challenge. She wanted everything else to be in place before she made herself a priority. Even finding the necessities—a good grocery store, dry cleaners, animal hospital, etc.—wasn't easy. Her lack of sleep began talking its toll, and she knew it was time to ask for help.

By the time Kathy found me, it was apparent that she needed a mild antidepressant and a prescription sleep aid to get through the night. Together, with the help of her physician, we recognized how sleep had become last on her list, and then she and I, as a team, reprioritized her time. We looked at how her stress was affecting her sleep and we developed new methods to decrease this stress. Over time the stress waned and she began working again from 9 A.M. to 3 P.M. when the kids came home. As she built a new network of business contacts and friends, and became more familiar with her surroundings, life got better. The balance she created in her sleep had an enormous impact on her quality of life. She was able to come off the sleep aid and eventually the antidepressant. As a sleep specialist, I know that lack of sleep can compound daily stress, while at the same time daily anxiety can impact sleep. So it's a vicious cycle. The secret is to find the vicious cycle's weak point and break it.

Anxiety and Stress: Sneaky Silent Sleep Killers

The inability to turn the mind off at bedtime and cage your worries and anxieties for the night is a leading cause of sleeplessness. Stress and sleep generally don't mix. All of us at one time or another have experienced the effects of angst, worry, nervousness, and even excitement on our ability to fall asleep fast and stay that way. Between 65 and 75 percent of patients I see in clinics have either anxiety or depression adding to their sleep problem, making these issues the largest component to most disordered sleep. Stress has become a natural aspect to daily living, and it's not something we can extinguish entirely from our lives. But there are solutions. The key is to learn how to manage stress so it minimally affects us.

QUIZ

1. Do you find yourself having racing thoughts at night once you have turned out the lights? Put another way: Do you have trouble turning off your mind?

This turns out to be one of the most common complaints I hear in the sleep clinic. Acknowledging having racing thoughts is an important part of identifying sleep problems.

If you answered yes, score +2 if this is a daily experience.

If you answered yes to experiencing this at least four out of seven days, score +1.

If you answered yes to experiencing this three days or less a week, score 0.

➤ Experiencing racing thoughts is quite common and you need to do something to distract yourself from thinking.

2. Do you have muscle tension in your shoulders, neck, and back?

Muscle tension obstructs the ability to fall asleep and stay asleep, and unless you pay close attention, it may be something of which you are unaware.

If you answered yes, score +1.

3. Do you find yourself sleeping less because you have too much to do?

This is a signal that sleep is not as important as it should be.

If the answer is yes, score +1.

4. Do you find yourself unable to get out of bed because you feel so tired?

This is a tough one because it can be a sign of depression, sleep deprivation, a biological rhythm disorder called phase delay, or a combination of problems.

If yes and you are not getting enough sleep, score 0.

If yes and you are getting enough sleep, score +1.

5. Have your friends told you that you seem "hyper" or "always so tired"?

Many of us do not even notice that our speech is rapid or slowed, our legs twitch, or that we are falling behind during activities where normally we would be at the head of the line. Listen to your friends and peers if they tell you these things, as they are certainly a sign of sleep deprivation and anxiety.

If you answered yes to either of these, score +1.

6. Do you find that your daytime sleepiness interferes with your productivity?

If yes, you are likely sleep deprived, as research shows that we are 40 percent less productive with even minimal sleep loss.

If you answered yes, score +1.

7. Do you find yourself highly emotional (angry at the kids or spouse, crying) when you have no real reason to be and it's not related to another condition, such as your menstrual cycle (for menstrual-related problems, see the quiz in the gender section, on pages 58–59)?

If yes, this is also a sign of both stress and sleep deprivation. It could be a sign of depression as well.

If you answered yes, score +1.

Scores:

If your score is 5–7, you guessed it: You are a cat on a hot tin roof. Follow the Action Plan below.

If your score is 3–4, then you may have some anxiety contributing to your sleep issues. Follow the Action Plan, anyway, but you may not need it at all.

If your score is 1–2, then it is unlikely that anxiety is your foe, but if you're close to answering positively to questions #1 and #2, then you may still want to consider the Action Plan below.

Action Plan:

If you answered yes to question #1:

❑ If you find that your mind simply will not shut off when you lie down at night, try counting backward from 300 by 3s. This is a difficult task, and will distract you from thinking about your other things.

❑ If you can't even get to the point of counting because you have so much on your mind, then consider a worry journal. This is where you write it all down so you can worry about it later. We will go into more detail on this idea later, in the 28-night program, but for right now, writing down a list is often helpful—getting your thoughts out of your head and onto paper, where you won't forget them.

If you answered yes to questions #1 and #2:

❑ If you are so overwhelmed by your thoughts and cannot conquer them, consider:

➤ Moderate exercise and stretching before bed. Although some argue that exercise can stimulate the body and prevent sleep, exercise can reduce anxiety in some people. So it might be a good idea to experiment with a mild to moderate exercise routine before bed. An evening, low-intensity yoga or meditation class is also an option.

➤ A hot bath or shower with aromatherapy (fragrant bath salts) and low lighting (no candles—fire hazard).

➤ A massage from your spouse or bed partner. Again, this is all about reducing tension.

➤ Watching TV (with headphones, so you do not disturb your bed partner).

➤ Reading material that won't get you thinking too hard or stimulate your mind too much.

If you answered yes to question #3:

❑ You need to sit down with yourself and whomever you live with and seriously consider your current responsibilities. You can't expect to "flip a switch" and fall into blissful sleep. You have to make time to wind down. Find a way to make sleep a priority. If nothing else, make one hour before bed your cut-off time. No matter what else still stands on your list of To Dos, once you're within one hour of going to bed, let everyone know you are down for the night. And stick to it—don't delay your bedtime.

❑ Try a hot bath or massage before bed here as well.

If you answered yes to question #4:

❑ Try making a list and organizing your time as best you can, and remember you are not super human and cannot get it all done in one day. Give yourself a reasonable task list, prioritize it, and then take the last three things off the list.

❑ Just how much sleep you are getting: Four hours? Almost seven (this is the average)? Eight? If you're not getting enough sleep, you probably know it. The 28-night program will help you get more quality sleep and, in effect, reduce your anxiety level overall. If you think you are getting plenty of sleep but still cannot get out of bed in the morning, then you really need to talk to your doctor about it. You could be suffering from depression or a sleep disorder. Keep reading, because both situations can be helped by the methods described in this book. (If you do seek treatment for, and are diagnosed with, depression, I urge you to use this book in addition to your treatment.)

If you answered yes to questions #5–#7:

❑ Try getting more sleep with one of the methods described above, and if it does not help, then you may need to seek further medical attention.

General Tips to Reduce Anxiety Before Bed:

- Hide illuminated clocks from view to avoid clock-watching during the night, as it can lead to anxiety over sleeplessness.
- Avoid eating within three hours of bedtime, as digestion can interrupt your ability to relax.
- Because alcohol, tobacco, and caffeine can exacerbate anxiety, avoid these before bedtime. Specifically, avoid alcohol and tobacco within three hours of bedtime, and caffeine within five hours.

Caffeine: The Robber Baron of Sleep

There's no denying that today's drug of choice is caffeine. It's the most widely used psychostimulant in the world. And in standard daily practice, about 85 percent of Americans use caffeine regularly, many to help bolster wakefulness in the morning or to stay alert throughout the day. There is no nutritional need for caffeine in the diet. Moderate caffeine intake, however, is not associated with any recognized health risk. We're willing to throw upward of five dollars over the counter for this drug in the form of a designer coffee. Every working day, Starbucks opens four new outlets somewhere on the planet, hiring 200 employees. But caffeine isn't ubiquitous due to popular coffee and tea hangouts; it's found in soft drinks, medicine (especially cold medicines and pain relievers), candy, ice cream and other desserts, and even water. (Yes, it's true. Some bottled water companies market "Java water.") Multiple sources of caffeine make it incredibly easy to consume, sometimes unintentionally. About 78 percent of us drink at least one cup or can of a caffeinated beverage daily, and 25 percent of us drink four or more cups or cans a day. In technical terms, our average daily intake is about 280 milligrams—or over 16 percent above the recommended daily allowance.

> How much caffeine do you ingest in a typical day? Turn to page 50 to tally up your milligrams. The National Sleep Foundation recommends less than 240 milligrams per day, which amounts to about two cups of regular coffee . . . but less than half of the jolt one popular coffee shop will serve you in their "medium"-size cup. If you're a soda fiend, roughly one six-pack will get your caffeine levels just over 240 milligrams.

Caffeine's effects on sleep are determined by a variety of factors, including amount, the time between caffeine ingestion and attempted sleep, individual differences in metabolism and sensitivity and/or tolerance to caffeine. People differ greatly in their sensitivity to caffeine; some people can drink several cups of coffee, tea, or soft drinks within an hour of sleep and notice no effects, whereas others may feel stimulating effects after one serving. Caffeine does not accumulate in the bloodstream or body and is normally excreted within several hours following consumption. (Caffeine can begin to take effect within fifteen to twenty minutes and reaches peak concentration in the blood in sixty to ninety minutes after ingestion, then gets metabolized in the liver. Complete clearance of caffeine from the body, however, doesn't occur until twenty-four to forty-eight hours after the last cup! Keep in mind that excretion rates vary from person to person based on age, weight, sex, hormonal status, and metabolism.)

Thus, there is no one grande mocha half-caf, fat-free fits-all set of guidelines for using caffeine responsibly. I love a good cup of joe myself, but I also know my limits. You, too, can get in tune with how your body responds to caffeine and can make adjustments so that it's less likely to disrupt your sleep.

> Some studies have shown that high doses of caffeine (200 milligrams or more) can increase anxiety ratings and induce panic attacks in certain people.

Caffeine does have its bonuses. It increases alertness, cognition, and shortens reaction time. It's been shown to relieve pain, thwart migraine headaches, reduce asthma, and elevate mood, as well as improve performance on many tasks. If you're an athlete or very physically active, you know that caffeine can amplify a workout or a high-intensity exercise performance. It can increase endurance, boost one's focus and, best of all, make a rigorous physical activity like running a marathon or cycling 100 miles feel a bit easier. Who wouldn't want such an endeavor to feel easier? Even a trip to the gym for an extreme exercise session on a Saturday morning to make up for a week of inactivity (a.k.a. "weekend warrior") will be easier with a cup of stimulating java beforehand. What's more, researchers are now suggesting that caffeine—specifically coffee—is associated with better glucose tolerance and a substantially lower risk of type 2 diabetes.

> Caffeine has been proven to enhance athletic performance in a variety of activities, especially running, swimming, and cycling. The consumption of just two cups of coffee can speed 1,500-meter running performances by four seconds and increase kicking speeds at the ends of 1,500-meter races by 3 percent. Other studies have indicated that caffeine can boost 100-meter swimming velocity and enhance sprinting ability on a bicycle.

But you know the downsides to caffeine: a possible increase in anxiety; physiologic effects like the "jitters"; stomach upset from the high acid content; and, most importantly for our purposes, it can disrupt nighttime sleep. Caffeine can reduce slow-wave (deep) sleep and decrease total sleep time. Individual sensitivity to this varies, and usually those most sensitive to caffeine's effects are acutely aware of it. However, because its effects are often underestimated once tolerance begins to develop, moderate, regular caffeine use in the late afternoon or evening is a frequently overlooked cause of one's complaints of sleeplessness. Therefore, you may not feel like the caffeine affects you since you can get to bed after having that cup of cappuccino, but it will still impact your sleep! Six eight-ounce cups or more of coffee throughout the day are likely to cause insomnia at night, even if not taken just before bedtime.

Studies looking at the brain have found that if you regularly use caffeine, and it's eliminated from your system, you will need it to function normally. Although the half-life of caffeine—the amount of time it takes the body to eliminate one-half of the total amount of caffeine consumed—is approximately three to seven hours, depending upon your individual metabolism, the effects may last as long as eight to fourteen hours. Several factors can lengthen caffeine's half-life, such as some medications, liver diseases, or pregnancy. The half-life of caffeine in pregnant women is eighteen to twenty hours; the half-life in women taking oral contraceptives is up to thirteen hours. Other factors, such as smoking and age, can shorten caffeine's half-life. For example, in children and smokers, the half-life averages about three hours.

QUIZ

1. Does even a small amount of caffeine make you jittery?
If a small amount of caffeine makes you "jittery" (i.e., small hand trembles, rapid speech, or a racing heart), you may have a caffeine sensitivity issue.
If you answered yes, give yourself 1 point (score +1).

2. Do you have a problem falling asleep?
Difficulty initiating sleep may be due to caffeine consumption late in the day.
If you answered yes, give yourself 1 point (score +1).

3. If you have had coffee in the day, when you wake the next morning, after having slept seven or more hours, do you feel like you had restful sleep?
Restful sleep after caffeine intake likely means that caffeine is either quickly metabolized or has little effect on you.

If you answered yes, then it is unlikely that caffeine has a large effect on you, so take 1 point away (score −1). If you answered no, then you are like the rest of us.

4. How many hours before lights-out do you have caffeine?
Greater than 5: score 0
3 to 5: score +1
Less than 3: score +2
If less than 3 and yes to question #1 above: score +3
Based on the half-life of caffeine, there are different possible recommendations for the general public.

5. How many hours after you wake do you have caffeine?
You may have a caffeine withdrawal problem.
Within one hour, score +2
Within two hours, score +1
Within three to five hours, score 0. (You may be experiencing the mid-morning lull.)

6. Do you feel like you need caffeine to start your day?
If yes, score +1
You may have developed a social habit as well as a physiological one.

7. How many beverages containing caffeine do you consume daily?
If greater than three, it's not about the taste for you (score +1).
If less than three, score 0.

Scores:

9–7: Java junkie. You may need a serious caffeine detox.
6–4: Caffeine is a likely contributor to your fatigue and possibly is causing sleep problems.
Less than 3: Caffeine likely has minimal effects on you.

How many milligrams of caffeine do you consume daily? This might be hard to calculate. Use the chart that follows to help make this guesstimate. You may find it helpful to start by categorizing your beverages based on your answer to #7: On average, how many eight-ounce cups of coffee, twelve-ounce glasses of caffeinated iced tea, and twelve-ounce glasses of soda do you drink a day?

_____ cups of coffee (including decaf, since it does contain trace amounts of caffeine)
_____ glasses of iced tea
_____ glasses of soda

Watch out for what a "cup" truly means. A large "cup" of coffee from most boutique coffee shops will pack a punch—providing five times the average amount of caffeine found in an eight-ounce serving of regularly brewed coffee from, say, your own kitchen's machine.

Now take your number of beverages and multiply them by their associated milligrams listed in the chart below. Add them up and you have a total milligram count of consumed caffeine a day.

Averages of Typical Caffeine Content in Popular Foods, Beverages, Medications

Product	Serving Size	Caffeine Content (mg)
Coffees		
coffee	8 oz.	110
Starbucks coffee, grande	16 oz.	550
espresso	1 oz.	90
instant coffee	8 oz.	75
caffe latte	6 oz.	90
Arizona Iced Coffees	8 oz.	40–50
coffee ice cream	8 oz.	58
decaf coffee	6 oz.	4
Teas		
Arizona Iced Tea, black tea	8 oz.	16
Arizona Iced Tea, green tea	8 oz.	7.5
*brewed, imported brands	8 oz.	60
*brewed, major U.S. brands	8 oz.	40
Lipton Brisk Iced Tea	8 oz.	6
Snapple iced tea, all kinds	8 oz.	21
Soft Drinks		
Mountain Dew	12 oz.	55.5

Product	Serving Size	Caffeine Content (mg)
Diet Coke	12 oz.	46.5
Coca-Cola	12 oz.	34.5
Dr Pepper, regular or diet	12 oz.	42
Pepsi	12 oz.	37.5
Diet Pepsi	12 oz.	36
7UP or Diet 7UP	12 oz.	0
Sprite or Diet Sprite	12 oz.	0
Caffeinated Waters		
Java Water	500 mL	125
Water Joe	500 mL	60–70
Chocolate		
Baker's chocolate	1 oz.	26
chocolate milk	8 oz.	5
chocolate-flavored syrup	1 oz.	4
dark chocolate, semisweet	1 oz.	20
milk chocolate	1 oz.	6
Medications		
Anacin	2 tablets	26
weight-loss products	2–3 tablets	80–200
Excedrin, maximum strength	2 tablets	130
Fiorinal	1 tablet	40
Midol	1 tablet	32
No-Doz, maximum strength, or Vivarin	1 tablet	200
Percodan	1 tablet	32
Other		
Sport Nutrition	2 tablets	200
caffeinated gum	1 stick	50
Red Bull	250 mL	80

*Tea can be difficult to approximate. How much you get out of a tea bag, for example, in one eight-ounce glass of hot water can vary significantly. Here's a breakdown of some common tea varieties (one tea bag) and their *approximate* caffeine content in milligrams:

black tea = 40 (but can range from 25 to 110 mgs)
oolong tea = 30 (but can range from 12 to 55 mgs)
green tea = 25 (but can range from 8 to 40 mgs)
white tea = 15 (but can range from 6 to 25 mgs)
decaf tea = 2 (but can range from 1 to 4 mgs)
herbal tea = 0

Action Plan:

I understand that it's nearly impossible, if not unrealistic, to cut caffeine entirely from your life. And I am not suggesting that you do. All I ask is that you use it responsibly. Here are some quick solutions to better manage intake:

Based on your answers to the quiz:

If on question #1 you scored +1, then if you've got to have a cup, try making it a small one with half decaf.

If on question #2 you scored +1, then try limiting your overall caffeine close to bedtime (you may require our caffeine cut-off technique described in our 28-night plan).

Other tips:

❑ Limit total caffeine intake to a maximum of 300 milligrams a day.

❑ Watch for hidden sources of caffeine, such as medications, chocolate, and frozen desserts.

❑ Avoid caffeine after 2 p.m., or at least try to reduce intake two to three hours before bedtime.

❑ If you need caffeine late in the day, try getting it from a source other than what you're used to and that is less potent, such as by drinking a cup of green or white tea in lieu of coffee. (Remember, tea can be potent, too, depending on type and strength of dilution.) If you must have the coffee, dilute the regular caffeine concentration by blending half regular, half decaf.

❑ Try the Caf-Nap. If you're really struggling to stay awake, drink a cup of java or black tea and then close your eyes and take a twenty-minute nap. When you wake up, the caffeine should be kicking in and you will have gotten some of your rest and will now feel energized for the remainder of the day. Avoid the caf-nap after 2 p.m. or it may prevent you from falling asleep that evening. (If you're very sensitive to caffeine and it affects you rather quickly—within too short a time period for you to rest—this may not be an option for you. The trick is to consume the caffeine quickly and then close your eyes while it gets absorbed and your body responds to it. This means you can't casually sip your

coffee over forty minutes and then try to lie down. Timing this
nap well is key.)

❑ If you have a frequent buyer's card at your local coffee shop, give
it to a friend when it is full.

You may also consider a caffeine cut-off point early in the day. The
28-night plan can help you wean yourself from caffeine and find the best
cut-off time for you. And be sure to bring your troubles up to your doctor. He or she may have some solutions for you based on your particular
body and lifestyle.

COPING WITH WITHDRAWAL

Caffeine withdrawal is very real—producing enough physical symptoms and a disruption in daily life to classify it as a psychiatric disorder.
Withdrawal from the drug produces a cluster of any of five symptoms in
some people:

1. headache (by far the most common symptom, affecting at least 50
   percent of people in caffeine withdrawal)
2. fatigue or drowsiness
3. unhappy mood, depression, or irritability
4. difficulty concentrating
5. flulike symptoms such as nausea, vomiting, muscle pain, and stiffness

The onset of caffeine withdrawal symptoms typically occurs within twelve
to twenty-four hours of stopping caffeine and peaks one to two days after
stopping. How long does it last? Anywhere between two and nine days.

What's considered excessive caffeine intake? Three eight-ounce
cups of coffee (250 milligrams of caffeine) per day is considered a moderate amount of caffeine. Six or more eight-ounce cups of coffee per
day is considered excessive intake of caffeine, which is approximately
500 milligrams. What was your total daily caffeine consumption in milligrams? If it was greater than 500 milligrams and you have sleep issues,
it may be time to cut back. As you begin to change *when* you consume

your caffeine so it doesn't interfere with your sleep, you may also need to cut back on *how much* you consume. And this is often the hard part.

➤ If you scored a 4 or more on the caffeine quiz, don't quit caffeine cold turkey! All this will do is throw you into a worse situation, with likely headaches, irritability, and being miserable. You'll also not sleep well during the caffeine withdrawal. So I repeat: Do not stop all caffeine. Use some of the techniques I explain to help reduce your caffeine intake and to drink responsibly.

A good way to cut caffeine intake without triggering serious withdrawal symptoms is by so-called **caffeine fading**. This is done by cutting down your consumption at the rate of one-half cup of coffee a day (or the equivalent of whatever form of caffeine you primarily consume). You can also reduce your intake by stepping down the number of total cups you drink a week. So, if you usually consume about eighteen cups of coffee per week, try to ax off two to five cups from your weekly menu. (If you are drinking more than ten cups of coffee a day, you should seriously consider cutting down.) Here's how to do it.

Consume caffeine regularly for a week while keeping a precise log of the times and amounts of caffeine intake (remember that chocolate, tea, soda beverages, and many headache pills contain caffeine as well as coffee). At the end of the week, proceed to reduce your coffee intake little by little by avoiding the equivalent of one-half cup of regular coffee a day. Remember to have substitutes available for drinking: If you are not going to have a hot cup of coffee at your ten-minute break, you might consider having decaf hot chocolate or herbal tea.

If possible, avoid using decaf coffee too much as a substitute, since there are healthier alternatives. Not only does decaf coffee retain its extremely high acidity, which can cause gastrointestinal problems, but the decaffeinating process itself typically involves solvents that are *possibly* carcinogenic (cancer causing, although the data is inconclusive). What's more, recent research has demonstrated that decaf might increase levels of fat in the blood—which, in turn, leads to a buildup of cholesterol.

Resorting to teas might be the better way to get that buzz without so much caffeine and acidity. True, tea has only half as much caffeine as coffee or energy drinks (or 40 to 60 milligrams per cup), but it's easier on the digestive system and can be a great way to minimize your caffeine consumption without feeling the effects of total withdrawal. Tea also has multiple health benefits. Along with trace vitamins and minerals, tea is rich in a class of disease-fighting antioxidants, which can help prevent cancer and heart disease. Tea has also been linked to dental health, aiding weight loss, boosting immunity, and increasing bone density. The bonus of tea is you have lots of tasty options since you'll find rows upon rows of different kinds of tea and flavors in your supermarket. And depending upon where you live, you may even be able to find a tea shop for more variety and high-quality teas. To decaffeinate your own tea, steep leaves for thirty seconds and then remove the water, which contains about 85 percent of the caffeine.

Another product gaining greater momentum in the market is Teeccino, a "caffeine-free herbal coffee," a blend of herbs, grains, fruits, and nuts that are roasted and ground to brew and taste just like coffee. You can likely find this product in a local natural food store and it might be worth trying. (By the way, "caffeine-free" and "decaf" don't mean the same thing. A caffeine-free product never had caffeine in it, whereas a decaf product started as one with caffeine and has since been processed to remove at least 97 percent of its caffeine.)

The Pluses and Minuses of Caffeine

Caffeine has mixed reviews in both the health and fitness world. Despite the potential negative—and often debatable—effects reported (e.g., raised blood pressure, increased heart rate, anxiety, headaches, heartburn, osteoporosis, birth defects, digestive ulcers, and so on), a lot of positive effects related to caffeine have been scientifically confirmed. We know caffeine can relieve fatigue, improve alertness and mental efficiency, creativity, and even improve athletic performance. Caffeine also has been shown to act as an antioxidant (stronger than vitamin C), and could protect against certain diseases, such as Parkinson's. So one can argue that, indeed, caffeine is a nonessential nutrient. Consumed in moderation (and at the right times of day), it can enhance your quality of life.

TRUE OR FALSE? SOME COMMON CAFFEINE MYTHS

Caffeine can cause relaxation. Answer: true. In smaller amounts, this has been shown to be true.

Caffeine use over time can lead to hypertension. Answer: false. There is no conclusive evidence to suggest that caffeine causes hypertension.

Drinking coffee can dehydrate you. Answer: false. In fact, drinking any hot liquid can cause dehydration because it raises core body temperature, which makes you sweat, thus causing dehydration. Caffeine is a diuretic, but there is a threshold level below which it has zero effect on fluid balance. It takes as much as 250 milligrams of caffeine in a single dose to have any diuretic effect, and even two cups of tea or coffee at once will have no effect on dehydration. But if you habitually have caffeine, your built-up tolerance is also a huge factor (not to mention the likelihood that you're *drinking* your caffeine with additional fluids to offset any diuretic effect).

Your Gender: Chrom X and (Not So Much) Y

As I mentioned in the first chapter, it's hard to draw definitive lines between men and women when it comes to sleep needs. But because men and women differ physiologically, it's no wonder that each sex has to deal with issues related to either the X or Y chromosome. Women, in particular, experience an enormous array of fluctuating hormones throughout their lives—from puberty to postmenopause—that coordinate complex and intricate brain and body changes. Men, on the other hand, have their own aging process to contend with, but experience less dramatic fluctuations in hormones that are likely to affect their sleep cycles.

For the purposes of this section, I'm going to focus on women and, in particular, on a woman who is *not* pregnant (pregnancy brings with it a host of sleep issues that go beyond the scope of this book). I'm also going to generalize the Action Plan by giving tips that can relate to both menstruating, perimenopausal, and menopausal women.

Approximately 75 percent of menopausal women experience hot flashes, a condition that can last for up to five years, and about 40 percent of menopausal women have sleep problems caused by them. Sleeping difficulties can lead to other problems, such as daytime drowsiness.

Women who suffer from serious PMS (premenstrual syndrome, which, in a severe form, is called premenstrual dysphoric disorder, or PMDD) have less slow-wave deep sleep—stages 3 and 4—during *the entire month*, not just during the premenstrual weeks. The most common PMS sleep complaints include all three types of insomnia (sleep-onset, sleep-maintenance, and early morning–awakening insomnias), hypersomnia (sleeping too much), unpleasant dreams and nightmares, and morning and daytime fatigue.

QUIZ FOR THE MENSTRUATING WOMAN

1. Do you experience a pattern of sleeplessness based on your monthly hormone cycle?

It's normal for the chemicals rhythmically coursing through a woman's body every month to impact her sleep.

2. Can you pinpoint certain weeks, such as the first, second, or third week leading up to menstruation, when it's more difficult to either get to sleep or stay asleep without being awakened in a cold sweat?

Alternating increases and decreases in hormones from day 1 of a cycle to day 21 and then menstruation can easily stir sleep problems, especially if you happen to be sensitive to one particular hormone. For example, the estrogen surge around day 12, which is right around ovulation, can be a source of sleeplessness. Likewise, the progesterone surge later on around day 21 can also cause problems, after which the decrease in both estrogen and progesterone can trigger awakenings. In fact, studies indicate that these lowered levels of estrogen and progesterone that spur menstruation increase nighttime awakenings and non-REM (NREM), or lighter sleep.

3. Are your premenstrual symptoms so severe, including fluid retention, bloating, cramping, and mood swings, that they impact your ability to get a good night's sleep?

All of these symptoms can naturally disturb sleep because they change your comfort level. What's more, severe PMS can change how much deep sleep you get, which affects daytime alertness and ushers in fatigue.

4. Do you find yourself more tired than usual just prior to or during your period?

Progesterone is a sleep-promoting hormone, and a decrease in progesterone is how your body triggers menstruation. If ovulation doesn't lead to a pregnancy, progesterone levels fall, making you more vulnerable to insomnia and other forms of disordered sleep.

QUIZ FOR THE PERIMENOPAUSAL AND MENOPAUSAL WOMAN

1. Are you in your late thirties and forties and suddenly experiencing insomnia?

Your symptoms of insomnia may actually indicate that you're beginning the transition to menopause, which is called perimenopause. From perimenopause through menopause, your ovaries gradually decrease production of estrogen and progesterone (again, this is a sleep-promoting hormone). The shifting of ratios of hormones can be an unsettling process, sometimes contributing to the inability to fall asleep. Also, waning levels of estrogen may make you more susceptible to environmental and other factors/stressors that disrupt sleep.

2. Have you had hot flashes that impact not only your ability to sleep soundly, but that change your breathing and snoring habits?

The hormonal changes going on that cause hot flashes can also prompt snoring for a variety of reasons (none of which are all that clear). In fact, nearly as many women snore as men by the time they go through menopause. One of the prime reasons for any snoring, however, is weight gain, which many women experience during menopause, and shedding a few pounds can help eliminate it.

3. Do your hot flashes make it very difficult to sleep even after you've cooled off and gotten comfortable again?

Hot flashes typically come with a surge of adrenaline that can take time to recede enough so you can settle back into sleep.

If you're a woman, chances are you can say yes to at least one of the preceding questions. If not, consider yourself lucky—your body must be so balanced that slight shifts in hormones don't affect you all that much. (And you probably haven't hit menopause yet.) Tips to dealing with changing hormones throughout life or within a monthly cycle can take up an entire book in itself. Instead of a concrete Action Plan here, I offer some simple solutions to minimizing the impact those occasional sleep-unfriendly hormones can have on you—no matter where you are in the arc of your reproductive body's life:

- Keep the bedroom cool.
- Avoid heavy bedding. No flannel or wool.
- Choose nightclothes that are very breathable: light cottons, sheer materials. Even during the winter, if you are prone to "power surges," then it may be okay to be a bit cold in the beginning of the night if it helps you stay asleep.
- Have a damp cloth near the bed so you can cool yourself quickly if you wake up feeling hot and sweaty during a week in your cycle when your hormones increase your body temperature. For women who experience hot flashes, a bucket of ice near the bed can come in handy.
- Change your nightgown if you wake up in a sweat, and keep an extra sheet on your side of the bed that can be removed once soiled.
- Use a sleep mask that you can place in the freezer to wear at night to keep cool.
- Try a cooling device that you wear around your neck to keep cool at a sports outing or while camping. Wear it at night. For safety reasons, make sure it's battery-operated and not attached to an electrical cord. Pillows that have a cooling effect while resting on them are also available now.
- If aches and pains related to your cycle prevent you from sleeping, try taking a mild, over-the-counter pain reliever or analgesic before going to bed. Just be sure the medication doesn't contain any stimulants. Popular drugs for combating menstrual-related ailments like bloating, backaches, headaches, cramps, and muscle aches contain caffeine.

- Discuss with your doctor any impact that hormone-replacement therapy (HRT) or birth control pills might be having on you if you take any of these drugs. Sometimes a tweak in the dose or a different pill entirely can limit sensitivity.
- Take naps on days when you feel extremely lethargic, which for many women is just prior to and at the start of their periods.
- Discuss your dietary supplement regimen, with your doctor. (More on supplements in Chapter 11.)

Taking Charge of Those Sleepless PMS Nights (If You Said Yes to Question 3 . . .)

- Consult with your doctor about increasing calcium and magnesium intake, both of which help the central nervous system and, in turn, PMS. Studies have shown a link between low magnesium and PMS symptoms.
- Consult with your doctor about taking extra vitamin B complex before and during your period.
- Drink lots of water. The more you drink, the more you flush through your system. Try to drink at least half of your body weight in ounces. So, if you weigh 150 pounds, drink seventy-five ounces a day (that's nine to ten glasses).
- Monitor sodium intake, which can retain fluids. Also monitor caffeine, alcohol, and carbonated drinks.
- Consider herbs and botanicals that assist digestion and urine flow—under your doctor's guidance. Diuretic herbs like dandelion and fennel powder, as well as juniper berries, ginger, chamomile, and lemon balm teas can also ease digestive and menstrual problems.
- Don't forget to exercise, even when feeling a bit uncomfortable during PMS. Exercise will help relieve cramps and bloating, and help you get a better night's sleep.
- Try some yoga, massage, stretching, and even acupuncture.
- Use a nonsteroidal anti-inflammatory like ibuprofen (Advil), naproxen sodium (Aleve), or aspirin to help alleviate muscle tension, aches, and pains. (Remember to ask your doctor if this is okay for you.)
- Make sure you get enough fiber in your diet, to prevent constipation. If you don't eat enough fiber-rich foods (which you should), try flaxseed oil or psyllium husks in a beverage. Remember that fiber works best with water.

A final item to note here about sleep problems related to the sex hormones is this: Not all disordered sleep during certain hormonal phases in a woman's life can be directly linked to hormonal issues alone. Other health problems can precipitate problems, which are then exacerbated by those hormones. For example, postpartum depression can cause disordered sleep that requires a unique course of action. Similarly, the journey through menopause can bring on a medley of emotional responses and mood swings. About 20 percent of women experience depression during this time frame, some cases of which have been linked to estrogen loss. Other causes can be blamed, however, such as life stress and coincidental social issues. A woman whose children are leaving the nest, who is retiring, moving to a smaller home, who has lost a spouse, or who is simply experiencing a "midlife crisis" confronts an enormous array of issues that can disrupt sound sleep and require more than the above-mentioned solutions. This is when speaking candidly with your doctor is an important part of maintaining your health and learning tricks tailored to your specific biological needs.

Hormonal and social issues combined are always at play. The best you can do is stay in touch with how your sleep is changed by your own cycle and address those areas where you know you need to take action.

As with gaining weight, craving peculiar foods, and preparing to lactate, disordered sleep is a pregnancy rite of passage. From the very beginning of conception to delivery, your body is under the spell of a growing fetus; everything from general anxiety, hormonal fluctuations, and physical discomfort can throw sound sleep out the window and leave you wondering when you'll ever return to a normal sleep routine. Many of the tips already mentioned can help you, but you may also find it valuable to ask your OB/GYN for specific tips throughout the course of your pregnancy as new complaints arise and old ones go away.

If you try any of the plans in this chapter, I encourage you to send me your feedback at www.soundsleepsolutions.com. Click on "Sleep culprits" and share your experience.

A final item to note here about sleep problems related to the sex hormones is this: Not all disordered sleep during certain hormonal phases of a woman's life can be directly linked to hormonal issues alone. Other health problems can precipitate problems, which are then exacerbated by those hormones. For example, postpartum depression can cause disordered sleep that requires a unique course of action. Similarly, the journey through menopause can bring on a medley of emotional responses and mood swings. About 20 percent of women experience depression during this time frame, some cases of which have been linked to estrogen loss. Other causes can be blamed, however, such as life stress and incidental social issues. A woman whose children are leaving the nest, who is retiring, moving to a smaller home, who has lost a spouse, or who is simply experiencing a "midlife crisis" confronts an enormous array of issues that can disrupt sound sleep and require more than the above-mentioned solutions. This is when speaking candidly with your doctor is an important part of maintaining your health and learning tricks tailored to your specific biological needs.

Hormonal and social issues combined are always at play. The best you can do is stay in touch with how your sleep is changed by your own cycle and address those areas where you know you need to take action.

As with gaining weight, craving peculiar foods, and preparing to lactate, disordered sleep is a pregnancy rite of passage. From the very beginning of conception to delivery, your body is under the spell of a growing fetus; everything from general anxiety, hormonal fluctuations, and physical discomfort can throw sound sleep out the window and leave you wondering when you'll ever return to a normal sleep routine. Many of the tips already mentioned can help you, but you may also find it valuable to ask your OB/GYN for specific tips throughout the course of your pregnancy as new complaints arise and old ones go away.

you try any of the plans in this chapter, I encourage you to send me your feedback at www.soundsleepsolutions.com. Click on "Sleep culprits" and share your experience.

much deep sleep you get, which affects daytime alertness and ushers in fatigue.

4. Do you find yourself more tired than usual just prior to or during your period?

Progesterone is a sleep-promoting hormone, and a decrease in progesterone is how your body triggers menstruation. If ovulation doesn't lead to a pregnancy, progesterone levels fall, making you more vulnerable to insomnia and other forms of disordered sleep.

QUIZ FOR THE PERIMENOPAUSAL AND MENOPAUSAL WOMAN

1. Are you in your late thirties and forties and suddenly experiencing insomnia?

Your symptoms of insomnia may actually indicate that you're beginning the transition to menopause, which is called perimenopause. From perimenopause through menopause, your ovaries gradually decrease production of estrogen and progesterone (again, this is a sleep-promoting hormone). The shifting of ratios of hormones can be an unsettling process, sometimes contributing to the inability to fall asleep. Also, waning levels of estrogen may make you more susceptible to environmental and other factors/stressors that disrupt sleep.

2. Have you had hot flashes that impact not only your ability to sleep soundly, but that change your breathing and snoring habits?

The hormonal changes going on that cause hot flashes can also prompt snoring for a variety of reasons (none of which are all that clear). In fact, nearly as many women snore as men by the time they go through menopause. One of the prime reasons for any snoring, however, is weight gain, which many women experience during menopause, and shedding a few pounds can help eliminate it.

3. Do your hot flashes make it very difficult to sleep even after you've cooled off and gotten comfortable again?

Hot flashes typically come with a surge of adrenaline that can take time to recede enough so you can settle back into sleep.

If you're a woman, chances are you can say yes to at least one of the preceding questions. If not, consider yourself lucky—your body must be so balanced that slight shifts in hormones don't affect you all that much. (And you probably haven't hit menopause yet.) Tips to dealing with changing hormones throughout life or within a monthly cycle can take up an entire book in itself. Instead of a concrete Action Plan here, I offer some simple solutions to minimizing the impact those occasional sleep-unfriendly hormones can have on you—no matter where you are in the arc of your reproductive body's life:

- Keep the bedroom cool.
- Avoid heavy bedding. No flannel or wool.
- Choose nightclothes that are very breathable: light cottons, sheer materials. Even during the winter, if you are prone to "power surges," then it may be okay to be a bit cold in the beginning of the night if it helps you stay asleep.
- Have a damp cloth near the bed so you can cool yourself quickly if you wake up feeling hot and sweaty during a week in your cycle when your hormones increase your body temperature. For women who experience hot flashes, a bucket of ice near the bed can come in handy.
- Change your nightgown if you wake up in a sweat, and keep an extra sheet on your side of the bed that can be removed once soiled.
- Use a sleep mask that you can place in the freezer to wear at night to keep cool.
- Try a cooling device that you wear around your neck to keep cool at a sports outing or while camping. Wear it at night. For safety reasons, make sure it's battery-operated and not attached to an electrical cord. Pillows that have a cooling effect while resting on them are also available now.
- If aches and pains related to your cycle prevent you from sleeping, try taking a mild, over-the-counter pain reliever or analgesic before going to bed. Just be sure the medication doesn't contain any stimulants. Popular drugs for combating menstrual-related ailments like bloating, backaches, headaches, cramps, and muscle aches contain caffeine.

- Discuss with your doctor any impact that ho therapy (HRT) or birth control pills might b you take any of these drugs. Sometimes a twe different pill entirely can limit sensitivity.
- Take naps on days when you feel extremely l many women is just prior to and at the start of
- Discuss your dietary supplement regimen, (More on supplements in Chapter 11.)

Taking Charge of Those Sleepless PM (If You Said Yes to Question 3 . .

- Consult with your doctor about increasing calcium an intake, both of which help the central nervous system PMS. Studies have shown a link between low magne symptoms.
- Consult with your doctor about taking extra vitamin B and during your period.
- Drink lots of water. The more you drink, the more you your system. Try to drink at least half of your body we So, if you weigh 150 pounds, drink seventy-five ounce nine to ten glasses).
- Monitor sodium intake, which can retain fluids. Also m alcohol, and carbonated drinks.
- Consider herbs and botanicals that assist digestion an under your doctor's guidance. Diuretic herbs like dand powder, as well as juniper berries, ginger, chamomile, balm teas can also ease digestive and menstrual prob
- Don't forget to exercise, even when feeling a bit uncon PMS. Exercise will help relieve cramps and bloating, ar a better night's sleep.
- Try some yoga, massage, stretching, and even acupun
- Use a nonsteroidal anti-inflammatory like ibuprofen (Ad sodium (Aleve), or aspirin to help alleviate muscle tensi pains. (Remember to ask your doctor if this is okay for
- Make sure you get enough fiber in your diet, to prevent you don't eat enough fiber-rich foods (which you shoul oil or psyllium husks in a beverage. Remember that fibe with water.

CHAPTER 3

The Three People Who Steal Your Sleep . . . and How to Manage Them

Think how rich you'd be if you could bottle that sensation of feeling like a million bucks in the morning, which all of us have felt at one time or another in our lives. Such a magic potion would surely make being an overworked parent, cohabitant of a restless sleeper, or frequent traveler a whole lot easier.

Meet Peter, a world-traveling businessman who had significant problems with his sleep.

Peter came to me as a friend and eventually became a patient. Peter's work schedule could be maddening. He is one of the top executives in his company, but his sleep issues developed long before his rise within the company. He started out in sales, which meant getting up early for breakfast meetings and staying late for client dinners. In between he was learning his product, checking his sales figures, reviewing his competition, and trying to stay awake. Peter found coffee early in his career and quickly progressed to being a two-cup morning guy, plus two cups at lunch and two cups in the afternoon. He attended client dinners about twice a week and at least one morning breakfast with either his boss or a new client. His wife was very understanding; she knew that if he wanted to get ahead at his job, he was going to have to put in longer hours than others. Peter would rush home to eat with the kids and put them to bed, and then he was right back on the computer with e-mails and research every night.

As the years passed, Peter moved up in the company and eventually had territories covering over half of the United States. This meant his travel was constant—he became a platinum club member almost overnight. By the time he reached me, his sleep schedule was in shambles and he was always fighting exhaustion. He was consuming a whopping eight to ten cups of coffee or some caffeinated drink per day, and drinking alcohol with clients over dinner before bed. He had gained about fifteen pounds and was accused of snoring.

Peter and I sat down and dealt with a few big topics to start. First, we looked at his sleep schedule and discussed how to regularize it. Next we looked at his travel schedule and worked on when he should fly and how his sleep schedule should be affected when traveling. Third, we developed an exercise program that he could use in his room to at least keep him moving while he was not at home. And finally we created a travel sleep kit for both the plane and hotel to help him when he was away. It took us almost three months to work on these stages, but as we put each piece into place, Peter started to notice a difference. He was not only less sleepy on a daily basis, but he noticed how much more productive he was when he slept more. He also started to lose some weight and was seeing his kids and wife more often.

What stunned Peter the most was hearing his boss ask, *What's your secret?* His boss had also noticed the positive changes. When Peter shared his experience, his boss wanted to visit a sleep specialist as well.

In this chapter, we continue our questionnaires and Action Plans by considering the other three people who take away from your sleep: you as a parent, you as a busy traveler, and your bed partner.

You as Mom or Dad: Balancing the Act Between Parenting and Sleep

Parents and caregivers get less sleep than other adults, and that's no surprise. About one-half of all parents have their sleep disturbed an average of twice a week because their child awakens them during the night. Parents of infants are awakened the most, and lose the most sleep; they are awakened an average of four nights a week, losing close to an hour of sleep each time.

In a child's first year of life, a parent loses more than 200 hours of sleep.

Even though the chance of a child disturbing your sleep wanes the older he or she gets (especially if you're a worrywart during those rebellious teen years), having to wait eighteen or so years to return to quality sleep would be a nightmare.

Insomnia is also a problem for parents and caregivers. Nearly three in ten experience insomnia at least a few nights a week; about one-half of these insomnia sufferers say their problem increased after they became a parent. The sleep habits of children have a direct impact on those caring for them. Parents that are twice as likely to say they sleep less than six hours a night have children who are not good sleepers. And in addition to not getting enough sleep, children's sleep habits cause moderate to significant stress on marriages and relationships, particularly for parents of infants and toddlers. No surprise there, either.

When asked how many hours of sleep they need per night, the majority of parents say they think they need between eight and nine hours of sleep. But parents of children ten years old or younger average about seven hours a night, and parents of newborns and toddlers get only 6.2 hours.

Books on sleep for children from infancy through the teenage years are abundant. So are books on sleep for adults. But what about *parents*? Is there any solution to surviving parenthood without accepting sleep deprivation? As a parent myself, I understand why the majority of parents would change something about their child's sleep if they could. But that's not always possible.

Maryann's Story

It's hard to tell the difference between "normal" sleep deprivation for a parent of a newborn and "abnormal" sleep deprivation that can lead to disaster. I was a new mom at thirty-two and just so excited to have a baby that I forgot to pay attention to my own sleep needs. About eight months into motherhood, I nearly fell asleep at the wheel after a quick trip to the grocery store. The close call scared me, making me wonder if this was every new mother's experience or just me. That's when my husband suggested that I ask my doctor for advice on getting more and better sleep. At the root of the problem was my baby's constant need for me. . . . She was colicky, temperamental, and not the best of sleepers. How was I going to deny my child what she wanted when she's so vulnerable and dependant in those early stages of life? My husband couldn't do much— after all, he wasn't the one breast-feeding and tending to the nighttime cries for food. I was the only one who could calm the baby quickly.

While my doctor said much of my experience was normal, he warned that if I didn't take better care of myself, I'd certainly have problems caring for baby Emma. I learned how to prioritize my daily tasks better so I wouldn't feel the need to do as much as I could—and I also learned to sleep when the baby slept instead of checking off my list of To Dos. The best piece of advice was teaching my husband how to respond to the baby so we could begin taking shifts. That way, the baby wasn't always reliant on me. And if she needed breast milk, we had some ready to go from a bottle so he could feed her, especially if it was in the middle of the night. This also helped him bond better with the baby. Emma is now eighteen months old, and my better sleep habits have given me more energy to be a happy mother *and* wife.

QUIZ

1. Are you woken up by your child, either crying or asking for something, more than once a night?

If yes, my next question is, are these legitimate awakenings or is your child manipulating you? (Legitimate intrusions are due to illness, special needs children, etc.) If, however, these are *not* legit, you and your spouse need to look at the issues and attack them with a plan together (see below).

2. Are these awakenings more than forty-five minutes into your sleep cycle (after you have fallen asleep)?

If yes, the damage is more severe because you may have gone into deep sleep. Your ability to awaken and be able to make good decisions is also decreased because you were likely in deep sleep.

3. Are you and your spouse discussing your children (good or bad) while in bed?

Studies show that having discussions on highly emotional topics (and we all know kids raise our emotions) can prevent sleep and even prevent deep sleep.

If yes, stop. This only aggravates your situation. Have these discussions out of bed in a neutral place.

4. Are you tired and do you feel un-refreshed in the morning?

If yes, and you get enough sleep and are not suffering from a sleep disorder yourself, then the kids are a possible culprit.

5. Are you getting angry/frustrated with your children around their bedtime? Do you have a hard time getting them to bed? Do they cause you to have increased stress and difficulty falling asleep?

If yes, it may be better to have a third party come in (i.e., a sleep specialist) or ask your spouse to step in, as you are likely going to spiral downhill.

You may have noticed that on this quiz I left off the scoring points. The reason is because answering yes to *any* of these is a likely cause of your sleep issues, so a score of greater than 1 means you need to consult my Action Plan.

Action Plan:

- ❏ Ask yourself: Am I a morning person or an evening person? How about my spouse? Based on your answer, learn how to take shifts. If you are best in the A.M., then take the 3 A.M. shift onward, and go to bed a bit earlier if possible (say 9 to 10 P.M.), while your late-night partner takes the 9 P.M. to midnight shift. (Hopefully no one is awake from 12 to 3 A.M., but if so, then again, split this up.) A few exceptions to consider:
- ➤ You may need to change this schedule based on commitments with work, social obligations, or if your child is ill.
- ➤ The person "on-call" may need to use a baby monitor on his or her side of the bed, and get up without waking the other person out of a sleep cycle.

➤ If it is not your shift but you wake up, do not open your eyes; maintain a relaxed state and try to return to sleep. Consider earplugs on your night off.

➤ If you are concerned about the other person's ability to handle the situation, discuss it with him or her during the daytime hours and create a list of situations in which you should be woken up—otherwise, your partner needs to figure it out alone.

In light of the findings from the 2004 "Sleep in America" poll, the National Sleep Foundation recommends the following for parents and caregivers:

• Make sufficient sleep a family priority. It's important for the health of *all* family members.
• As parents, you need to determine the amount of sleep each family member needs and take steps to ensure individual needs are met.
• Establish regular bedtime routines, creating a quiet and comfortable bedroom. Televisions and computers need to be out of the bedroom, and caffeine should not be part of a child's diet.
• Learn to recognize sleep problems. The most common sleep problems in children include difficulty falling asleep, nighttime awakenings, snoring, stalling and resisting going to bed, having trouble breathing, and loud or heavy breathing while sleeping. These sleep problems can be evident in daytime behavior such as being overtired, sleepy, or cranky.
• Talk to your child's doctor about sleep—even if your doctor doesn't broach the topic.

A SPECIAL NOTE ABOUT KIDS CRAWLING INTO YOUR BED

Although most books on children's sleep recommend that the children do not sleep in your bed, I disagree in some cases. Every family's situation will be different, but some circumstances can call for a parent to share the bed with a child. If your sleep is consistently disrupted based on putting your child back to bed several times each night, then it's okay to consider letting him or her in your bed—but for a limited time. As an example, if Little Suzie sneaks in a 4:30 A.M., then go ahead and let her stay, especially if she (and you) can fall back to sleep easily. If she can't get to sleep, then she must be put back in her own bed. Over the course of the following few weeks, reward your kids for staying in their bed longer and longer.

More on this topic in the next section.

Your Bed Partner: One Bed, Two Sleepers

If you're not sleeping well with your bed partner, you are not alone. It's a big problem—so bad that nearly 25 percent of partnered adults frequently sleep alone. Whether your partner snores loudly, tosses and turns violently, or simply has a different sleep cycle that doesn't coordinate well with your own, dealing with a bad bed partner can be a challenge. Sleep, however, is related to marital satisfaction; in fact, researchers are now studying how curing sleep problems leads to marital bliss. At the Sleep Disorders Center at Rush University Medical Center, scientists are evaluating the impact of sleep disorders—particularly sleep apnea—on marital satisfaction and whether or not treating more cases successfully can affect the divorce rate. In general, couples with lower marital satisfaction are more likely than their counterparts to report symptoms of insomnia and daytime sleepiness, and they're getting less sleep than they did five years ago. And if you've got children adding to your problems, well . . .

> The average person changes position forty to sixty times a night, which can cause your partner to move, too. In terms of the clock, sleep disturbances amount to nearly an hour of stolen slumber each night.

> One of the loudest snores recorded in *Guinness World Records* was 93 decibels (120db is a jet engine), by Kare Walkert of Kumla, Sweden, in 1993.

QUIZ

1. Does your bed partner sleep with a light on? Including TV or a reading light?
   Yes   No

2. Does your bed partner listen to music or TV when trying to fall asleep?
   Yes   No

3. Does your bed partner snore?
   Yes   No

4. Does your bed partner like it hotter or colder than you?
   Yes   No

5. Does your bed partner like a firmer/softer mattress than you?
   Yes   No

6. Does your bed partner smell to the point of keeping you awake?
   Yes   No

7. Does sex prevent you from falling asleep?
   Yes   No

8. Does your bed partner wake up at a different time and not let you get back to sleep?
   Yes   No

If you answered yes to more than two of these questions, you may have a situation where your bed partner is affecting your sleep.

Action Plan:

If you answered yes *to:*

Question #1: Light is a possible problem. Solutions to consider:

❑ Use an eye mask for less illumination.

❑ Have the bulbs by the bedside or over the bed replaced with forty-watt bulbs.

❑ Consider a screen light reduction (you can find these for computer screens where the glare is reduced by placing a film over the screen).

❑ Ask your partner to use a small book light instead of relying on a larger bedside or overhead light.

❑ Switch sides of the bed if you face the light your bed partner is using.

❑ If light is coming from the window, consider blackout shades or dark fabric.

❑ Use light-tight strips on the rims of doors.

❑ Make a pillow barrier. A wall of pillows can help dampen sound and movement from your partner.

Question #2: Noise is a possible problem. Solutions to consider:

❑ Earplugs. Get the kind that are "NLR" (noise level rated). The best you can get with earplugs is a reduction in sound level of about thirty-three decibels. That's because even with your ear canals completely blocked, the bones in your head will conduct sound to your inner ear. Snoring rarely exceeds eighty-five decibels, so that means you can reduce it to around sixty-two decibels—about the sound of a normal voice during the most intense snoring. You can find lots of snoring relief kits online, or at your local pharmacy. Check out http://earplugstore.com for its snoring relief kit.

❑ A white noise machine/CD. Numerous types are available. The key is to find a sound that is soothing to you. Many companies provide sampler packs, which you can test out to determine what will work best for you. Marpac, for example (www.marpac.com), is a company that specializes in "sound conditioners" that drown out noise; you can program the machine to provide what you want to hear, such as surf, rain, waterfall, brook or lake shore, or country eve. A cheaper alternative is to set the tuner of your FM radio between any two stations. The pseudo white noise you'll hear will do wonders to mask unwanted sounds. Ceiling fans or stand-alone fans can also provide a constant hum similar to white noise that can be sleep-friendly. But if the air they blow is bothersome, these are not a good idea.

❑ Combination earplugs with white noise. New earplug technology utilizes sound-dampening earplugs with a white noise emitter. You can also find devices that allow someone to watch TV with earphones while the other person sleeps.

❑ Consider pillow speakers, which are mini-speakers that deliver private, directed sound to just one listener. They can be plugged into the mini-jack of any standard CD player, radio, or similar unit. You have many brands and styles from which to choose. Retailers from RadioShack to Sharper Image carry them, or you can go online and Google them. I suggest the stereo speakers (so there will likely be two or one long one; and I have not yet found ones that are wireless).

Question #3: Noise is again a possible problem, albeit a bit more serious since snoring can be a sign of sleep apnea. This is a potentially life-threatening disorder that can be causing daytime sleepiness, heart problems, and concentration and memory problems. If the snorer stops breathing, a telltale sign of sleep apnea, he or she should visit a sleep specialist. Snoring, however, isn't always attached to a sleep disorder. If the snoring doesn't make the person tired the next day, you can do a few things short of sending him or her to an ear, nose, and throat (ENT) surgeon.

❑ Try nasal decongestants. These will reduce inflammation and allow for wider breathing passageways.

❑ Consider "breathe-right" strips (these tend to work only for those with a narrow nose and should be properly placed about 1.5 centimeters above the tip of the nose).

❑ Think about the possible impact of allergies. Look at pillows, sheets, fabric softeners and detergents, pets in the bed, dust, mold, perfume, and so on, that can affect the bedroom environment. All of these can cause congestion, which can worsen snoring.

❑ Think about alcohol consumption, which often worsens snoring.

❑ Think about weight issues. Consider losing five to eight pounds, as research shows that this can help reduce snoring significantly.

Question #4: Temperature is a problem. While a comfortable room temperature is around seventy-two degrees Fahrenheit—when you're awake—the ideal sleeping temperature is slightly cooler—between sixty-five and seventy-two degrees. The reason is that a mild drop in body temperature often induces sleep, which is why lying in a cool bed after a hot bath is so relaxing. Temperatures above seventy-five or below about fifty-four can disrupt sleep. Too many blankets can also interrupt your sleep, as you'll need to be able to move freely. Tips to dealing with temperature sensitivity:

❑ Consider an electric blanket for only one side of the bed, or a comforter with half down and half cotton.

❑ Consider a fan for one side of the bed, or a window only open on one side.

❑ Make sure the colder person has warmer pj's—this can help quite a bit.

❑ Consider socks and a nightcap for warmth (most heat is lost from the head).

Question #5: Differences in mattress preferences are more serious than people think. Quality mattresses are a big expense for many, and their impact on our sleep is underestimated. It's not so hard, however, to find the perfect mattress setup that addresses both bed partners' needs. It's crazy to think that two people who have a seventy-five-pound weight difference require the same sleep surface in terms of firmness and support. Differing sleep positions are also part of the equation. Some solutions:

❑ Obtain two twin mattresses of differing firmnesses and band the beds together for intimacy. Two twins roughly equal a king, and you can connect the two "customized" twins using a pad that rests along the junction of the two, then top it off with one mattress pad. What you get is "independent suspension."

❑ Review some of the more high-end mattresses that offer adjustable sides to the bed. Some mattress companies will even tailor-make a mattress based on you and your bed partner's specifications. Some also employ certain design elements that dampen any movement of your partner so that he or she doesn't wake you by turning over or getting out of bed.

Refer to Chapter 4 (page 111) for tips on selecting a mattress.

Question #6: Odor can be more problematic than you might think—and it's a sensitive subject. Many people will come home from working late, eat a quick bite, and jump into bed without a shower. Then they sleep while sweating all night. The average person sweats nearly four gallons a month while sleeping, causing an odor in the sheets and sometimes the mattress itself. Body odor and breath are also influenced by diet, no matter how good one's personal hygiene is (see box). Some solutions:

- ❏ Review your partner's evening diet, alcohol and caffeine consumption, and bedtime hygiene.
- ❏ Request bedtime showers. Take them together for increased intimacy.
- ❏ Consider a stronger mouthwash and toothpaste.
- ❏ Enforce better gum care via dental floss or tape, and a powerful toothbrush such as an electric one.
- ❏ Consider a new mattress that targets your problem. Simmons, for example, has a HealthSmart mattress designed to wick away sweat and moisture with a removable top for washing germs and odor out (see Chapter 4). If firmness is an issue, there are several companies that have adjustable firmness levels or will actually determine what your needs are.

Body odor is not just genetic. Diet and body odor share a strong direct link. Given the hundreds of millions of dollars spent each year on personal care products and deodorants, it's surprising that few people acknowledge the role that a change in diet can have on reducing body odor. The following are foods that can influence body odor: red meat, overly processed foods such as those made with refined white flour, added sugars, hydrogenated oils, and foods high in preservatives and chemicals. Certain "healthy foods" can also increase body odor, such as garlic, onion, and exotic spices. Conversely, some plants actually act as deodorizers, namely parsley, cilantro, celery, and all mint species. The aromatic herbs are also excellent deodorizers: sage, rosemary, thyme, oregano, and so on.

Question #7: This one is a bit controversial. Anecdotal evidence shows that men seem to get sleepy while women are more energized after sex. If you're the one who feels energized after sex, planning this activity around sleep is not always a good idea.

Question #8: Not everyone hits the hay or wakes up at the same time. With different work schedules, social schedules, and general lifestyles, couples typically need to go to bed and wake up at different times on different days. But just because one person goes to bed or wakes up does not mean the other must keep the same timing. The trick is to maintain separate bedtime and waking schedules without either one disturbing the other's sleep.

❏ Discuss the issue with your bed partner. If you prefer to continue sleeping while your bed partner gets up, convey to him or her what you need to stay asleep and not be awakened. Similarly, if your bed partner is the first to go to bed, find out how you can best slip into bed without waking him or her or interrupting his or her sleep cycle. You may, for example, need to use a dim night-light for navigating the bedroom so you don't crash into furniture and make a lot of noise. I have even seen slippers with little lights on them to help guide you around a dark bedroom.

❏ For the one who gets up first, try pillow speakers that plug into an alarm clock or a vibrating alarm clock so the person still asleep is not disturbed.

❏ Restrict fluids. If you usually wake your partner (or vice versa) as you get out of bed to use the bathroom, try not to drink any liquids within two hours of bedtime.

❏ Consider sleep aids. If you or your partner has sleep problems, see a specialist and consider the appropriate use of sleep medications.

NOTES ON OTHER POTENTIALLY BAD BED PARTNERS: PETS AND CHILDREN

Let's take a moment to discuss further the issue of kids (plus pets) in the bedroom, which I touched upon briefly in the Mom & Dad section. This issue can go much deeper than just Little Suzie hopping into your bed on occasion and for a limited time period in her life. Entire schools of thought are devoted to the idea of "the family bed" or "co-sleeping." If you're ever interested in learning all you can on this topic, you'll find volumes of information and viewpoints in other books and on the Internet. Much of this subject matter revolves around cultural differences. And because pets are also considered members of the family to many people, they, too, sometimes get a spot on the bed. Is this all okay from a sleep doctor's perspective?

I have several thoughts in this area. I personally have had pets in our bed, kids in our bed, and I've certainly heard both sides of the story. In contemplating the issues as well as the pros and cons, here are my simple rules on the subject:

1. Everyone has a different tolerance level for these types of situations, so both bed partners must agree on who gets to sleep where. If kids and/or pets don't disturb anyone's sleep, then there's usually no harm.

2. Understand that once you allow kids and/or pets to share your bed, it becomes difficult to curb or stop the habit. Kids and pets rarely understand moving from a family bed setting to their own bed. I usually suggest a separate bed for kids so that they know and understand that they have their own space, thus promoting their independence and teaching them how to fall asleep on their own. As previously mentioned, however, many children naturally go through phases when they are very young wherein they climb into your bed in the middle of the night. And that's usually okay.

3. When drinking alcohol, no one should allow a child or pet in the bed. Studies have shown that this is when problems occur, such as children getting hurt, pushed off the bed, smothered, etc.

4. Make sure that your intimacy needs do not suffer from sharing your bed with kids and pets. Remember the bed is for both sleep and sex; do not trade one for the other.

5. Have your allergies checked. Over time, it's quite easy to develop allergies to pets and not realize it. If you wake with a stuffy nose every day, put Fido or Fluffy in his or her own space. A recent study demonstrated that a reasonable percentage of pet owners who allow their pets in bed have sleep problems.

6. Review the habits of the pet and/or child to make sure they are compatible with you: A snoring bulldog or a child who likes to sleep horizontally instead of vertically can be a bigger problem than you might think. Consider training your pet to sleep in his own bed next to yours if Fido tosses and turns.

Final note: The issue of children (and even pets) in the bedroom constitutes its own book. It's a huge topic that I cannot possibly address completely in this book. It's also a difficult topic to approach in a broad manner and apply to everyone's unique situation. If this is a subject area that concerns you and your family, you should seek guidance starting with your family doctor, pediatrician, or veterinarian.

You as the Busy Business Traveler: Stress, Performance, Jet Lag, and Other Business Demands

Business travel and sleep have to coexist or you'll be far less productive than you may think. Yet there's a catch-22: You need quality sleep to function at your best, but you also need to get the most out of a business trip, which often cuts into time to sleep. Business travel demands high performance amid stress, hectic schedules, heavy meals, and late nights—all a recipe for poor sleep. Add shifting time zones, the dramas related to airports, hotels, business dinners, convention duties, and whatnots to the mix . . . and you've got yourself a recipe for guaranteed sleep deprivation. (See Chapter 11 for more tips on coping with traveling.)

More of us are traveling for business today than ever before. We're also traveling for pleasure, and even mixing business and pleasure travel on occasion. We naturally fall out of our sleep routines when we're away from home, and many of us have difficulty sleeping in a different environment (called the "first-night effect"). What's more, we're likely to experience the "on-call effect," or the inability to maintain sleep while anxiously awaiting the next day's events (and that wake-up call). This is partly why my work with hotel chains has been so important (see www.crowneplaza.com, and click on The Crowne Plaza Sleep Advantage™). I've been helping the industry adopt better practices, specifically with regard to fine-tuning their rooms to attract sleep- and business-minded travelers. By installing superior mattresses and offering bedside sleep amenities, hotels can ensure their customers get the best night's rest for an optimal day's work.

About three in ten people admit to missing work, events/activities, or to having made errors at work because of being too sleepy or having a sleep problem. More than half of adults have been late to work due to sleep issues.

The on-call effect is when you have trouble sleeping because your mind is literally "on-call" as it anticipates the need to be alert and awake at some point in the near future. For physicians, it's waiting for the phone to ring and to respond to an emergency; for new parents, it's waiting for the baby to cry and to attend to it; and for travelers, it's awaiting the dreaded wake-up call.

QUIZ

1. How many days per week do you travel? (Score +1 for every day traveled, so if you travel three days per week, you get +3 points.)

Traveling on a weekly basis is more likely to have effects on your sleep than only a couple of times a month.

a. Does this require air travel?

If yes, see questions b, c, and d.

Travel by air can affect your sleep because of the crossing of time zones, but travel by car can be more dangerous if you are sleep deprived.

b. Does this require crossing time zones? (On average, more than two?)

If yes, add +1 per time zone crossed.

Crossing more than one time zone can lead to feelings of jet lag even if you never get on a jet.

c. Does this require an overnight stay?

If yes, deduct −1 for each day you stay overnight in the same time zone.

If you get a chance to stay overnight, then your body will have the time to adjust to the new time zone.

d. Do you go multiple places?

If yes, add +1 for each new place you stay. (For example, let's say you travel from Atlanta to L.A., stay for one day, and then fly to Chicago. Your score would be calculated as follows: +3 (3 zones) −1 (stay overnight) −1 (fly back a time zone to Chicago) +1 (multiple sites) = 2 points.

Multiple stays usually mean extra stress.

2. Do you find yourself worrying about the wake-up call?
If yes, score +1.
You may experience the "on-call" effect described earlier.

3. Do you find yourself uncomfortable sleeping in an unfamiliar environment?
If yes, score +1. If you get better sleep away from home, score −1.
If you have a hard time sleeping in strange places, you may be experiencing the "first-night effect," a frequently observed phenomenon whereby people sleep less efficiently than usual on the first night of several successive nights in a different or new environment. If it is just the opposite, then it's your home environment that may be preventing you from having a good night's sleep. Check out my suggestions in Chapter 4.

4. Does your trip require entertaining guests and with this drinking alcohol?
If yes, and it's more than you usually drink, score +1.
Alcohol is known to make you fall asleep faster, but will disrupt your sleep architecture.

5. Can you nap on a plane?
If yes, this can be helpful, but will not likely affect your score.
You may be able to reduce your fatigue with a quick nap. Try a Caf-Nap, detailed on page 53.

6. What is your diet like when traveling? Different? Healthier? Fattier? Heavier?
If yes to anything but healthier, score +1; if you eat better on trips, deduct −1.
Most people tend to "cheat" on their typical diet, resorting to fast food because they don't have the comforts of home and a kitchen. With restaurant or fast food, there's much less control over ingredients.

In addition, if they are sleep deprived when traveling, research shows that people tend to eat higher carbohydrates and sweets than normal. (See Chapter 5 about weight loss and sleep.)

7. Do you have time/energy to exercise while traveling?
If yes, and you do exercise, score −2.
This is a great way to help reduce the symptoms of jet lag, help with sleep, and increase your metabolism to burn off those extra calories.

8. Do you find traveling stressful?
If yes, score +1.
We know that stress can increase restless sleep.

Scoring:

If you scored more than three points, you likely experience transient sleep disturbance whereby traveling has a negative impact on your sleep habits, causing sleep deprivation. You should pay greater attention to practicing better traveling habits so you remain as alert and refreshed on trips as you are when you're working from your main (home-based) office. Many people have good sleeping habits until they travel.

If you said yes to any of the questions above, the following Action Plan consists of tips from a journey's start to finish that you'll find helpful for getting the most out of your trip without sacrificing precious shut-eye.

Action Plan:

Preparing to Travel:

❐ Get a good night's rest before your travels commence (this may mean starting to plan and pack for your trip two days in advance to avoid the last-minute rush the night before). Also eat well and exercise the day before, as this will give you an edge and ease troubled sleep during your trip.

❐ Increase your water consumption. Drink as much as you can.

❐ Create a travel sleep kit (see page 85 and Chapter 11).

❐ Wear something comfortable, loose-fitting, and layered. You never know if it will be too hot or too cold on the plane, train, or other form of transportation.

❐ Avoid red-eyes or nighttime flights. If an overnight flight is unavoidable, ask your doctor about a short-acting sedative to help assist your sleep.

❐ Travel business or first class, if possible.

❐ Expect travel delays—*before* you travel! A lot of the frustrations related to travel today are beyond your control, so you have to just let it go. Have good reading material or a portable listening device on hand for those unexpected delays.

If you feel obliged to work on your laptop, make sure it's juiced up with a charged battery.

En Route and During Your Travels:

❐ Try to power nap on the plane and schedule your flight during your afternoon lull. This is when having a C-shaped pillow that fits around your neck is helpful, as it keeps your head from bobbing around or you getting a stiff neck. Take off your shoes or at least loosen the laces to improve circulation.

➤ Seat selection: Sitting in the middle of the plane will provide a less bumpy ride. Try staying away from the galley and the bathroom due to traffic and odors. If you are more than six feet tall, consider an aisle so you can stretch out. Windows are also good for leaning your head and pillow against. Usually bulkheads are reserved for those with mobility issues or families with babies (you will want to steer clear of them). For more tips on seat selection, go to my Web site.

❐ Hotel and room recommendations: Try to revisit the same hotels and even stay in the same room. Maintain consistency with a particular brand (of hotels). Ask for rooms away from the street, sources of light, garbage bin, elevator, stairway, ballroom, conference room, nightclub/bar or restaurant, elevator, and ice machine. Inquire about "quiet floors" or designated noise-free areas, and also ask about sleep-friendly amenities such as blackout curtains, night-lights, and a menu of pillows.

❐ Utilize your prime time. If you're on a two-to-three-day trip that crosses multiple time zones, try to plan meetings on your home time's midday hours, because your body will not have enough time to adjust.

❏ Avoid making critical decisions or attending important meetings on the first day after arrival. Avoid driving long distances on the first day after arrival.

❏ Let the sunshine in. During the day and meetings, let as much light into the room as possible and stay active, whether talking or just taking notes.

Food and Fitness:

❏ Watch your diet during your travels. Eat meals in the right time zone. On the first day, the right zone is approximately thirty minutes to one hour earlier or later (early if you travel west, and late if you travel east; this will change based on the duration of your stay until you catch up to the time in your destination place). For example, if you fly from New York to Los Angeles (five hours, with three time zones), when you arrive in L.A. at 10 A.M. from an 8 A.M. EST flight, it's really lunchtime for you. Wait about an hour and then have a "late" lunch. On the next day, have lunch at 11 A.M.; on the following day, have lunch at noon. Consider taking supplements and vitamins if you don't have total control over what you're consuming and know that you'll lack in the nutrient category.

❏ Ask your doctor if a supplement like melatonin is okay for you and how you should use it safely. Keep in mind, however, that many general physicians are not well-trained in the use of melatonin. While it's an over-the-counter product that doesn't require a prescription in the U.S., you should not try it without speaking with your doctor first. (More on melatonin in Chapter 11. The National Sleep Foundation also provides excellent information on this unregulated supplement. Go to www.nsf.org.)

❏ Monitor alcohol and caffeine consumption. Restrict nicotine. Nicotine can keep you up and awaken you at night; it can stay in your body for as long as fourteen hours. It should be avoided particularly near bedtime and if you wake up in the middle of the night.

❏ Exercise on the road. Utilize hotel gyms or go for a walk first thing in the morning.

❐ When your body wants to be asleep but you want to be awake, go out in the bright sunlight or engage in some physical activity.

❐ Relax before bedtime. Stress not only makes you miserable, it wreaks havoc on your sleep. Develop some kind of pre-sleep ritual like reading, light stretching, or taking a hot bath to break the connection between all the day's stress and bedtime. These rituals can be as short as ten minutes. You're bound to have more time on the road for this type of activity than at home where you might have other responsibilities pulling at you.

YOGA ANYWHERE YOU GO

Try the following two sequences before bed the next time you're in a hotel room. (If you have neck or back problems, consult your doctor or chiropractor first.)

Sequence 1:

- Sit cross-legged on the bed with your back straight but relaxed. Hang your head forward so your chin rests on your chest for a few seconds. Then, slowly drop your head back as far as you comfortably can and feel the stretch. Repeat five to six times.
- Take your left ear down toward your left shoulder. Hold for a few moments. Bring your head back up to center and do the same thing on the right side. Repeat on both sides.
- Turn your head slowly to look over your left shoulder and back as far as possible. Return your head to center and repeat over on the right side. Do this back and forth for five to six times.
- Drop you chin to your chest and slowly rotate your head in a clockwise direction. Then go counterclockwise. Repeat these rotations two to three times.

Sequence 2:

- Lie down with a pillow under your head for support; hands are by your sides, palms facing up.
- Close your eyes and focus on your breathing, paying close attention to your exhalations. Feel your abdominal muscles expanding as you breathe in.

- Scan your body mentally and find any tense or tight areas. Release that tension.
- Take in a deep belly breath through your nose that fills your lungs from the bottom up. Hold your breath as long as you can.
- Open your mouth and exhale dramatically, squeezing out all the air. Then, inhale again through the nose as deeply as you can. Hold the breath for several seconds.
- Exhale again out the mouth with noise (like a sigh) if you wish. Let it all out.
- Mentally scan your body once more, letting go of any leftover tension.

Crossing multiple time zones can play funny games with your circadian rhythm. If you are traveling from New York at 8 A.M. to California and it's a five-hour flight that crosses three time zones, that means you land at 10 A.M. L.A. time. But it's really 1 P.M. "your time" back in New York, and making an 11:00 A.M. meeting in L.A. works out great. Consider the reverse, however: Say you leave L.A. at 5:30 A.M. to get to New York for a 1 P.M. meeting in downtown Manhattan. If getting up that early is not normal for you, try to take a nap on the flight so you're refreshed by the time you land in New York. Or leave later in the morning from L.A. and schedule the meeting for *the following day* so you have time to adjust.

How about setting your body clock to a new time zone *before* the journey? By using light box therapy and techniques to induce sleep, you can reset your circadian body clock before a journey, thus preventing jet lag from the very start. If you are planning a trip across more than two time zones and want to get accustomed to your destination's time zone quickly, this might be an approach to take.

Let's say you have an important business trip for which you have to fly east. Before flying, you'd go to bed and wake up earlier each day while using the light box (that you can rent or buy; check out www.litebook.com) in the morning and winding down earlier in the evening. If you're traveling west, you would expose yourself to bright light later in the day, go to bed later and wake up a little later in the morning.

Using a light box allows for more concentrated, intense light (higher "lux," and at the right wavelength) than sitting in front of your bedside lamp. You'll learn about lux, a measure of light intensity, in Chapter 4. In terms of health and well-being, our bodies respond to a specific combination of light wavelengths that happen to be identical to the peak wavelengths of sunlight. If you do not have the time or inclination to get a light box, then consider direct sunlight as the next-best alternative. Light boxes, while producing artificial light that mimics the sun's intensity, don't emit ultraviolet radiation. They are designed to produce those perfect wavelengths of light (peaking in the optimal "blue" wavelength range, or 460 nanometers) and the light gets directed angularly at your eyes for the greatest effect.

The Traveler's Survivor Kit

earplugs
eye covers
favorite soothing music and headphones or a device like an iPod
C-shaped pillow that fits around your neck

It's been proven that sleep inspires *insight*. By restructuring new memory representations, sleep facilitates the extraction of explicit knowledge and insightful behavior. Translation: Sleep keeps you smart, thinking on your toes, and creative and able to process and manipulate information quickly. Losing as little as one and a half hours for just one night reduces daytime alertness by about one-third. Imagine what this means if you miss two hours of sleep while journeying across the country on a red-eye from San Francisco to Boston for an important meeting that you have to lead first thing in the morning.

If you can shift your body clock naturally prior to departing, this can be a particularly useful technique if your business trip doesn't allow for much time to adjust before kicking into high gear and demanding your top performance.

Try and switch over to your new time zone right away by going to bed and getting up at the same time you would normally, but on this new time zone. So if you usually go to bed at 10 P.M. in L.A., do the same the first night you land in New York even though your body might think it's only 7 P.M. Then, the next morning, try to go for a walk outside, exposing yourself to light and movement that can help reset your internal clock.

CHAPTER 4

The Extreme (but Easy!) Bedroom Makeover

When's the last time you considered the look and feel of your bedroom as a possible source of your sleep problems? Sleepless nights aren't all about your body and what's going on inside your mind. Your bedroom is a big part of the equation.

You're about to kick-start a transformation of your bedroom that will take it from a place where you sometimes sleep . . . to a sanctuary for relaxation and luxurious slumber. I'm going to make this simple, fun, and exciting to do. You're going to evaluate what you've already got. You're going to find the trouble spots and tend to them. And, best of all, you're going to give yourself permission to spend some money. A little money goes a long way when it comes to giving your bedroom a much-needed face-lift. The room not only benefits; *you* are going to feel and see the results, and it won't take long.

Unlike a bustling kitchen, which in many homes is often the center of activity and people gathering, your bedroom should conjure sleep without much effort. Think about that for a second: When you enter your bedroom, does it instantly relax you? Or does it feel like any other room in the house? Or, worse, does it fill you with anxiety because it reminds you of sleepless nights? Let's see if we can't fix that.

In early 2006, a new study survey showed that American adults struggle with their resolutions to lose weight, get more sleep, and stop smoking. In fact, the poll, conducted by the Wall Street Journal Online and Harris Interactive Health-Care (a market research firm), revealed surprising results: Only 11 percent of Americans make a New Year's resolution to get more sleep. And of those who do vow to get more sleep, only about a third (32 percent) succeed. I wonder, however, how many of those who didn't succeed never made physical changes to their bedroom setting as a first step. . . .

SHUTTING THE DOOR TO THE REST OF THE WORLD

Being a master chef is often dependent on access to the finest and freshest ingredients, certain know-how, and a well-equipped kitchen in which to practice with skill and precision. The same goes for becoming an expert sound sleeper. You will need an individualized recipe with ingredients that include: a great mattress, appropriate lighting, sound, setting, and so on, as well as the knowledge to practice good sleep habits on a routine basis. It's not just about how to count sheep or mold your pillow around your head. You must create the optimal sleep environment first and then you'll be surprised by how other sleep-promoting practices begin to fall into place.

Today too many of us allow the outside world to intrude upon our bedroom. Everything from television watching, chatting on the phone, answering e-mails or surfing the Internet, to arguing with a spouse or child. When these things become bedroom activities, we lose that image of our bedroom being a true sanctuary. Instead, it becomes much like any other room in the home, and can no longer immediately make us feel calm, tranquil, and ready for bed. No wonder so many of us have a hard time getting to sleep.

Have you ever treated yourself to a day spa or weekend spa resort? If so, then you've probably experienced a "quiet room," a space reserved only for one "activity": lying down in the luxury of silence amid dim lighting with nothing to distract your senses. In the quiet room there's nothing in particular to watch, nothing to touch other than the softness of your lounge chair; nothing to taste; nothing to hear but maybe soothing white noise; and nothing but a fresh, clean scent in the air. The challenge, then, in this room is staying awake! It's much too easy to fall asleep and feel wonderful doing it. Now what if you could create that same scenario at home—without having to go to a spa? If you do want to go to the spa and do these things, I give you both the permission and prescription to do so. Just tell them, "This is what my sleep specialist ordered."

It's time to take a good look at your current bedroom setup and make a few changes. And the best way to do this is to go step-by-step through the five senses.

Many people have a television in their bedrooms. The topic has gained attention recently with regard to children's bedrooms, which have become media centers instead of sleep centers. Nearly one-third of preschoolers and even 20 percent of infants and toddlers have a television in their bedrooms. Children with a television in their rooms go to sleep almost twenty minutes later and sleep less than those without a television, a loss of more than two hours of sleep a week. This has also been correlated to obesity in children. And just because a television in a child's bedroom has such effects doesn't mean adults can't experience the same consequences. (On the flip side, I've had patients who require the television to fall asleep; if they didn't watch television to distract themselves, they wouldn't fall asleep until at least an hour or more after their normal bedtime. So for adults, the TV question varies, which we'll revisit during the 28-night program.)

An in-depth consideration of the five senses is a great way to evaluate your bedroom and create the ideal sleep environment. The senses do have an order of priority, however, based on how much of an effect they can have. They are as follows, from what I feel is the sense with the greatest impact to the sense with the least:

1. sight
2. sound
3. touch
4. smell
5. taste

Sight

What we see significantly affects how our other senses process information and respond. Sight directly affects the circadian pacemaker, which is your biological clock telling you what time to sleep and what time to wake. In other words, what you see (both in content and brightness) can reset your biological clock and mean the difference between being blissfully asleep at 3 A.M. or wide awake staring at the clock. There are three areas to consider: light, color, and clutter.

Grab a pen and write down the answers to these questions:
How light is your bedroom?
   a. Nightstand bulb wattage: _____ (If you do not have a nightstand bulb, go to question b.)
   b. Overhead bed lights (recessed lighting, fan lights, etc.) wattage:
   _____
   c. Is there a TV or computer monitor in your bedroom? Is it on during the evening?
   d. Does your bed partner use a small reading light?
   e. How many windows are in your bedroom?
   f. Which direction do they face?
   g. Does the sun ever come directly into the room?
   h. Are there lights from outside your window, such as streetlamps, apartment building lights, or city lights?

Light meters: You can buy a light meter that measures your ambient light in either foot-candles or lux. Look for cheap, portable, handheld devices at camera and photography shops, or try an online distributor. You don't need anything fancy, so try to find one under $100. If this is not feasible, you'll have to estimate your bedroom's brightness given some basics of light exposure.

Proper placement of your bed should take the windows and any streaming light from natural (i.e., the sun and moon) to unnatural sources (lamps and streetlights) into consideration. You'll also want to limit the total wattage of light you have in your bedroom at night. During the evening hours, try to have no more than a total of 200 watts of light on, and while you're trying to wind down for sleep, be sure no one source of light emits more than forty watts. Once the lights are out and you're trying to sleep, there should be no more than five to ten watts of light on from all light sources (e.g., night-lights, closet lights, and so on).

What's a "Lux" of Light?

Light intensity (quantity) is measured in foot-candles (candela) in the United States, while it's measured in "lux" in most other countries. (A foot-candle equals about 10.74 lux—or, for a rough conversion, multiply foot-candles by 10 to get lux.) Most Americans are familiar with watts which are units of measurement for *electrical power*—and not necessarily light *intensity* (although higher outputs of electrical power correlate to brighter light emission). This is why we have the lux system to help us define intensity or brightness; it specifically measures how much light falls on your eyes. The human eye can adapt to a light intensity that ranges from 100,000 lux (brightest full daylight) down to 0.00005 lux (starlight). One lux is the illumination cast by a wax candle. A forty-watt bulb is about fifty lux. And a moderately lit bedroom measures around one hundred lux. Some other points of reference:

- Sunlight on an average day ranges from 32,000 to 100,000 lux.
- Traditional light boxes provide 10,000 lux (bright light therapy typically means greater than 2,500 lux; some light boxes are rated at 5,000 lux and are still very effective when they produce light with a peak in the effective wavelengths of 465 nanometers).
- Nighttime events in an outdoor stadium are approximately 1,400 lux (or 2,000 lux in front of goals).
- A bright office has about 400 lux.
- Moonlight represents about 1 lux.
- Starlight measures a mere 0.00005 lux.

Remember: A measurement of lux also depends on the distance between the light source and your eyes.

Here is what I want you to do:

- Strategically arrange the bedroom furniture around any incoming light and noise. If, for example, you share a wall with the laundry room in your apartment building, avoid placing the bed up against that wall. Avoid placing the bed directly across from a window that faces east (or you will be rising with the sun). If you can get away from the noise, but that puts you in the light, move away from the noise and buy some blackout shades.

- Replace high-wattage bulbs with low-wattage bulbs. Replace your switchers with "dimmers." Aim to reduce the total "time-for-bed" wattage in your bedroom to forty-five watts or less.

- Make sure your windows are covered. Consider blackout shades or heavy drapes to cover windows. These can also dampen sounds. Don't forget to use a drape clip, which will securely close the two sides of the drapery. (Try starting out by using a "chip clip," which works great. Chip clips are those huge clips sold to securely close bags of potato chips and other goods sold in large bags.)

- Eliminate computers and televisions from the room, and if that's not possible, use screen covers that reduce the glare that monitors and screens give off. (I found some great ones at www.sleeplamps.com.) Or just turn them off. If you must keep your CPU on, use a piece of black electrical tape to cover the little green light on the front of the monitor.

- Have a reading lamp or book light available for the one who wants to read before going to bed. (I like the Itty Bitty book light, but you'll find many to choose from. Go with what you like.)

- Use night-lights for hallways and bathrooms. These should emit low-level ambient light and be placed along a pathway to the target restroom. (Sleeplamps.com carries one that emits 0.5 watts.) You can also find directional night-lights that only point downward, which is also an excellent alternative.

- Keep eye shades in your bedside table. There are about twenty different kinds on the market so see the box for some things to think about.

Grab that pen again and answer this:
What colors dominate your bedroom?
Conventional wisdom aside, a recent analysis of color found that there is no direct relationship between colors of the environment and emotional states. There is, however, evidence that certain colors may

evoke a sense of spaciousness or confinement. Spaciousness appears to be attributed to brightness of color. And emotional responses to color are culturally learned.

The Cloak of Darkness: Eye Shades

What you want to think about:

1. Material: Make sure it's soft and that you're not allergic; silk and satin are my favorites.
2. Size: Make sure it adequately covers your eyes entirely so that no light can peek in.
3. Weight: If it's too heavy, it will rub against your eyelashes and this can be distracting.
4. Smell: Some now have aromatherapy built in, which can be fine or a bit strong; use milder scents like vanilla or rose.
5. Filling: There is everything from a mask that you can cool (a blue gel mask) to buckwheat, but there is no data to suggest one is better than another. If a traditional mask does not work for you then try some of these on for size.

What are some of these learned associations?

Cool Colors = those that evoke images of pastoral landscapes and ocean vistas. They are taught to elicit feelings of peace, tranquility, and relaxation:

Blue: peace, tranquility, calm, stability, and harmony. We can learn that blue conjures images of the ocean and sky. It may actually slow the pulse rate, lower body temperature, and reduce appetite.

Green: nature, environment, health, good luck, renewal, youth, and spring. Green's cool quality soothes, calms, and has great healing powers (a reason why it's often worn in operating rooms by surgeons).

Violet: relaxation, calm, mysticism, and eroticism. Lavender and lilac also fall into this category. Purple tones are often seen in children's playroom and bedrooms.

Warm Colors = those we can associate with images of heat, like fire or sunshine.

Red: danger, energy, love, desire, speed, violence, anger, emergency, exit signs, stop signs. Red can evoke a fight-or-flight response, raise blood pressure, and make the heart beat faster.

Yellow: joy, happiness, optimism, idealism, imagination, hope, sunshine, summer, gold, as well as decay, betrayal, and hazard. For some, yellow is too bright a color to have a calming effect in the bedroom.

Orange (a combination of yellow and red): balance, warmth, vibrance, enthusiasm. Orange is considered a warm color, like red, but to a lesser extent; orange expresses energy. Because it is demanding of attention, it's been used on caution signs.

As you can deduce, based on your culture, you want to stick with cool rather than warm colors. But also understand that you may react differently to certain colors, and you might have to experiment with an assortment of colors to find out which ones put you most at peace in your mind. (The same goes for your bed partner.) Neutrals such as pale gray, taupe, and beige exude restfulness and can be good choices for the bedroom, specifically because they are not particularly bright. Earth tones are gentle and will keep a bedroom feeling warm and snuggly, as long as you pay attention to the exact tones you use (two different beiges can evoke two entirely different feelings). Avoid bright white, which tends to be very stark and unsettling. Also avoid high-gloss finishes. Consider a matte or a flat finish. In addition, consider painting your ceiling something other than white. Remember: What wall are you probably going to see the most *from bed?*

Got cold feet? If you have a tile or hardwood floor in your home and it's wintertime, getting out of bed in the middle of the night can be quite cold and stimulating. Get a nice pair of slippers (I've even seen ones with built-in night-lights!) to put beside your bed or get area rugs to keep your feet warm and cozy. The color of your flooring can also have an effect on you. Deep rich woods may be more inviting to you than white or marbled tile. If carpeting is dominant, then pick muted colors and off-whites.

Besides the color of your walls, whether it's paint or paper, what covers and hangs on your walls also affects you. For example, imagine having a photograph that stirs negative emotions in you, for whatever reason. If this is the last thing you look at before going to bed, then you may have some unsettling sleep. Be careful how you decorate your bedroom. You know yourself best when it comes to choosing friendly, calming, and peaceful designs. I often recommend black-and-white photos, or color photos from fun family vacations or pictures of people you really enjoy being with. As for art, consider calming pieces like nature photography, landscapes, or images that put you at ease.

What Mood Is Your Bedroom?

Does the color of your bedroom make you happy, sad, calm, or excited when you enter it? Is it cozy and welcoming or stark and uninviting? If you were to give one word to describe how your bedroom colors make you *feel*, what would it be? If it's not calming, relaxing, soothing, sleepy, or something that you think promotes sleep, look around and think about what you would need to do get to one of those words. Remember, if red or orange calms you, then consider one of those colors. Just be careful not to make it too bright.

Finally, don't forget the color of your sheets and bedcovers. Bright oranges, reds, and yellows, while fun, may not send the message to your brain to go to sleep. Pick soft pastels, off-whites, and earth tones for sheets. Designs are fine, but make them subtle, not obvious. If florals are your favorite, again make the colors and designs relaxing to your eye.

Keep It Out of the Bedroom

An untidy room doesn't evoke peace and serenity. It can have a psychological effect on you, or keep you up at night worrying about cleaning it up as soon as possible. Keep your bedroom free of excess clutter, such as stuff you don't need lying on or around your nightstand, books stacked high, children's toys scattered about, or piles of mail, laundry, or furniture crammed together. You want to create an area that your eye views as flowing and positive. You want to avoid an area that signals stress, like bills to pay or laundry to do. Have you ever heard of a sanctuary with a pile of dirty underwear? Make keeping your bedroom in order a priority—more so than you view keeping your kitchen or living room in order.

Q. I hear a lot about feng shui. What is it and what's so great about it?

A. Feng shui (pronounced *fung shway*) literally means "wind" and "water." It refers to an ancient Chinese practice of creating balance in the placement of objects so that chi—the universal life force or energy present in all things—can flow freely. Although feng shui has been around for centuries, it's been all the rage in interior design and decorating lately. Applying its lessons to your home—specifically the bedroom—can indeed help you attain a more peaceful, sleep-friendly environment. Feng shui honors clutter-free rooms whose physical elements are harmonized perfectly in the space to support balance of mind and spirit to those who enter. You'll find lots of books on feng shui to help you design and colorize your entire home according to its principles. For the interior decorating enthusiasts or those who face problematic bedrooms with regard to arrangement, this subject is definitely worth investigating. You'll find many books on feng shui in any bookstore, and if you ask around friends and family, you probably have at least one self-proclaimed feng shui expert in your circle.

Sound

Sound rings in as the second most important variable to creating an ideal sleep environment. Grab a pen and answer these questions. If you want to, write the answers in this book!

How noisy is your bedroom?
Here are some things to think about.

  a. If you have a television in your room, do you or your bed partner sleep with it on? How loud is it?

Non-snorers who sleep with a snorer can lose an average of one hour's sleep per night. They also wake up, at least briefly, more than twenty times per hour during the night, producing fragmented and unrefreshing sleep.

  b. Does your bed partner cause any noise from snoring, teeth grinding, talking, or moaning during sleep? (Remember: The majority of Americans live with someone who snores, which can have a dramatic impact on quality and quantity of sleep for all people within earshot.)

  c. Does the house have noises that keep you awake, such as creaking floors or noisy air-conditioning/heating systems?

  d. What about the opposite: Is your house *too quiet*, in which case it elevates your anxiety level?

  e. Are you kept awake by other house members, such as children, newborns, or animals?

  f. Do external noises disrupt you, such as loose parts on your house's exterior, crashing branches, city noises, neighbors, or your neighbor's barking dogs?

  g. Do you or your bed partner use an alarm clock?

How to control noise levels (many of these suggestions were covered in Chapter 3):

- Consider music: nature and ocean sounds can help with relaxation and sleep.
- Consider a relaxation CD. (You can download my personal favorite at my site, www.soundsleepsolutions.com, for free when you register for my newsletter.)
- Consider white noise machines. Some companies specialize in "sound conditioners" that drown out noise. Or you can use the old trick of setting your radio between stations and keeping the volume low to create your own white noise!
- Consider earplugs.
- Consider a system for the television and any other device emitting sound. Earphones, pillow speakers, and a TV timer (for both light and noise) are options.
- With all of the preceding options, remember to keep the volume down, below 4 on most TVs.
- Check your alarm clock: If you and your partner wake at different times, consider a vibrating alarm clock that fits in your pillowcase so it doesn't disturb your partner. Or attach your pillow speakers to the alarm clock for your ears only.

What's in a Decibel?

People confuse decibels all the time, because they aren't "units" per se. A decibel is literally one-tenth of a bel—the number of bels (named after Alexander Graham Bell) being the common logarithm of the ratio of two powers. In other words, they measure a ratio of powers. Decibels do measure loudness, but it's best to think of them in terms of percentages because they aren't quantities of anything.

    0–the softest sound a person can hear with normal hearing
    10–normal breathing
    20–whispering at five feet
    30–soft whisper
    50–rainfall, refrigerator, large office
    60–normal conversation
    70–Some research suggests that any sound above this range can
       stimulate the nervous system.
    70–95 garbage disposal
    75–85 flush toilet
    80 doorbell; ringing telephone
    80–90 blender
    85–heavy traffic; noisy restaurant
    110–car horn; baby crying; shouting in ear; power saw; leafblower
    120–thunder
    170–shotgun
    180–rocket launching from pad

Remember, it may not be the decibels of the sound but the *content* that can keep you up. Whether or not you fall asleep easily to the sounds of a crying baby depends on your emotional attachment to that cry.

Window makeovers are also an option, especially if you live on a busy and noisy street. You can redo your windows by installing impact-resistant panes that absorb outside noise as well as block 99 percent of ultraviolet light. They also have the added bonus of being energy-efficient. These specialty windows have a plastic film, which acts as an insulator, inserted between two sheets of glass. Acoustic thermal pane windows will also do the trick.

If entire window makeovers are beyond your budget right now, consider window treatments geared for cutting down noise, plus light and heat in many cases. For example, Hunter Douglas is a company that makes window treatments and rates window coverings for sound. Another company, the Warm Co., in Seattle, sells "Warm Window" insulated shades that can reduce noise and light and prevent heat loss through the window.

SIGHT AND SOUND: THE ALARM CLOCK

Your alarm clock may end up being one of the most important purchases in your bedroom, and here's why: You really shouldn't need one. If you're well rested and your circadian rhythm is on cue and working with your schedule, you should be able to look at your clock and know when your body is going to wake you up. Now this may not always be the case, because special occasions will happen when you may need to wake early (e.g., to catch a flight, arrive early to work for a meeting, attend to children on Christmas morning, etc.). But for the most part, the true test of having a healthy sleep-wake cycle is in not having to rely on an alarm clock.

Keeping this in mind, you'll want a clock with the following features:

1. An LED light (of the time) that you can turn on and off. Once you know the time for bed, you shouldn't need it anymore throughout the night (unless an emergency wakes you up).

2. An adjustable volume control for the alarm.

3. Possibly the ability to have music or a CD/MP3 player so you can wake to the sounds of your choice.

4. A headphone jack, so you can attach pillow speakers or a vibrating device to wake you and not your bed partner.

Because staring at the time as you try to go to sleep can actually counter your attempts to fall asleep, you'll see later, during the 28-night program, that you should avoid having your alarm clock in view once you've hit your bedtime. This will also prevent you from getting riled up if you wake up in the middle of the night and can't get back to sleep easily.

Touch and Temperature

How you feel physically while in the comforts (hopefully) of your bedroom has a major influence on your ability to sleep well. Here are some questions to ask yourself:

- How hot or cold is it in your bedroom? As noted in Chapter 3, the ideal sleeping temperature is between 65 and 72 degrees— leaning more toward the lower temp. A room above 75.2 degrees Fahrenheit can cause restless body movements, nighttime awakenings, and less dream sleep; a room below 53.6 degrees Fahrenheit can increase the time it takes to get to sleep, and can cause unpleasant dreams.

- What season of the year is it? Your room needs to be cooler in the summer and warmer in the winter. If it's a dry winter, a humidifier can help; likewise, if it's a humid summer, an air-conditioning system can remove the stickiness in a room, or you may choose to invest in a dehumidifier (especially if you live in a coastal town).

- Do you sleep with the windows open or closed? This affects temperature.

- Do you take a bath or shower before bed? If so, this can raise your core body temperature, which might be quite helpful for falling asleep. Beware of using the bathroom attached to your bedroom for nighttime showers if it increases humidity levels too much.

- Do you exercise before bed? This, too, can increase your core body temp and induce sleep. (More on this topic in Chapter 6. Exercise is a powerful copartner with sleep, but timing when to exercise in relation to bedtime usually requires some experimentation. You'll get a chance to test this out during the 28-night program.)

- What materials make up your bedsheets, blankets, and comforters? Types of fabrics, from cotton to wool and polyester blends, can have a big impact on your ability to get comfortable or not.

- How often do you wash your sheets? What kind of detergent do you use?

- How old are your pillows and mattress?

- How hard or soft is your mattress? Do you like the feel of your mattress? Does your bedmate?

THREADING THROUGH THE MYTH OF YOUR SHEETS

A 250 thread count or 500? Egyptian cotton or pima? Bedsheets come in a staggering variety of sizes, fibers, weaves, colors, and styles. And you'll find a vast array of selections at both high-end retail stores and lower-priced outlets. The way bedding companies and designers market their products these days, it's no surprise we're all confused about what really makes a soft and cozy sheet set. They like to tell us what we need and hope we assume they're right. But does dishing out mega bucks for a sheet set really get you the best night's sleep?

For the most part, the answer is no. Thread count has become more of a marketing gimmick than a true indicator of quality. Some thread counts are false claims. The right way to count is to add up all vertical and horizontal threads in a square inch of fabric. Two hundred is typical; 400 may provide a finer, softer sheet. Above 400, the only difference is likely to be price. ("Percale" on the package means the sheet has a thread count of 180 or higher.)

1-2-3's of Picking the Best Sheets

1. Choose the fiber: For easy-to-care, comfy, and durable sheets, 100 percent traditional cotton remains your best choice. If you demand that your sheets look their best and you don't want to iron, look for cotton-polyester blends. Don't write off cotton blends, because they can be processed and finished to feel like butter. Take your time to feel the actual sheets when you go shopping. Don't just read the outer packaging and make a quick decision. Avoid buying based on price tag, the label, or what the salesperson pushes. Here's the decoder of fibers you'll likely find when you hit the linen departments:

   Egyptian cotton: Cotton cultivated in Egypt feels softer than other cottons, generates less lint, and is more durable.

   Pima cotton: Previously called American-Egyptian, this is a high-quality cotton developed from Egyptian cotton and that is grown only in the southwestern United States. The cotton is exceptionally soft, and the fibers are strong and firm.

   Modal: A category of manufactured fibers known for their strength. The fabric retains its shape well.

Lyocell: A manufactured fiber made from trees. It's soft, strong, absorbent, and wrinkle-resistant. It's also strong when wet and simulates silk or suede.

Polyester: The most common polyester for fiber purposes is polyethylene terphthalate, or PET. It's a strong synthetic fiber that resists shrinking, stretching, mildew, abrasion, and wrinkling. It washes easily and dries quickly. (Extra tidbit: It's also used to make plastic soft drink bottles.)

2. Any thread count between 200 and 400 is perfectly fine. Above 400 and you're likely wasting your money.
3. Make sure you buy sheets that match your bed size. Measure your mattress's thickness before you go shopping. (Place a stiff piece of cardboard between the mattress and box spring. Then place a piece of cardboard on top of the mattress. Now measure the distance between the two pieces.) Some mattresses can measure up to twenty inches thick.
4. Choose a fitted sheet that has elastic *all the way around* and not just at the head and foot. A fitted sheet should encase the mattress and grip all four corners with just a bit of room left over.
5. A note on color: Darker sheets will fade over time. They also show stains and hair (think of your pet pooch here) more readily than lighter shades. Also remember that the color can set the mood of the room. Lighter shades will make you feel cleaner, but stark white may change the feel to a hospital. Try cream, off-white, or pastels.

Keeping your sheets washed will help maintain their soft feel against your skin, as well as their clean scent. (Remember: Odor can impact falling asleep.) Depending on how much you (and your bedmate) sweat and release oils, you may have to adjust how many times a week you change soiled sheets for fresh ones. Change your sheets a minimum of once a week if you feel you or your bed partner are normal sweaters. If more than normal, then change twice a week. For best results, wash sheets in hot water; use a water softener if you have hard water. Avoid using bleach since it can break down the finer fabrics. For the many people who have skin allergies, using a non-dye, hypoallergenic detergent is likely the best way to go. When considering the no-dye formulas, try something scented—as long as you are not allergic to whatever they use to scent the detergent. Or test out some linen sprays on your skin and find a pleasant one that your skin won't react to. There are many sprays and aromatherapies on the market. There is evidence to suggest that some smells can cause a relaxation effect. You can find many of these products in stores at the mall (e.g., Bath & Body Works) or check out specialty stores online like Bloominggrove.net. Washing will affect your sheet's wear and tear, but they are likely to become even softer over time with every wash.

The High-Techs of Bedroom Accoutrements

It's been estimated that people spend more than $14 billion a year on retail sleep products. Because no two sleepers are alike, there's a big market for customized "dual comfort" sleep products to match personal preferences, especially for couples who try to sleep with each other. It's been amazing to watch the boom in sleep products, thanks to technology and companies dedicated to innovation. We now have beds that have individually controlled air chambers as well as memory foam that conforms to the body without generating too much heat. A company called Split the Sheets makes flat and fitted sheets that are divided down the middle to "split" the needs of two temperature-sensitive sleepers. One side is made with Polarfleece; the other is made with a light cotton. The matching pillowcases are lined with the same two fabrics on opposing sides. The Chillow is a pillow that keeps your head cool and can help relieve headaches, sunburns, hot flashes, or just be used as a regular pillow.

Hybrid comforters are also available. Select Comfort, for example, makes one that's thin on one half and thick on the other. Sunbeam manufactures a heated mattress pad with twenty temperature settings for each side.

And let's not forget about the flourishing mattress industry. The old-fashioned mattresses we used to jump up and down on as kids are a thing of the past. Now we have movement-absorbing mattresses that reduce the transfer of motion. (See my section on mattresses on pages 111–115.)

At some point in the future, we might be able to invent devices that accurately track our individual sleep cycles and wake us up at the perfect time. I have not used any of these devices yet, but the SleepTracker, which was named one of the best inventions of 2005 by *Time* magazine, sounds intriguing. This device uses sensors that detect motion and in turn your body's sleep stages. Basically, you set a window of time for waking up in the morning and when you begin to stir during that time frame, which typically correlates to when you're coming out of deeper sleep and toward wakefulness, it sounds an alarm to gently wake you. You wear it like a wristwatch, and it looks similar to sports watches. Axbo is yet another sleep phase alarm clock developed in Germany.

The sky's the limit in the sleep retail market.

PILLOW TALK

An old, deflated pillow can ruin a good night's sleep just as much as a bad mattress. Besides your mattress, which is the most important part of a good night's sleep, pillows are the second most important ingredient. It's not unusual to wake up with a sore neck and back because of your pillow. The most common problem is a pillow that's too stiff. People tend to buy pillows that are much stiffer than what they need. Particularly if you sleep on your back or your stomach, you will want a softer pillow, so that your head is not unnaturally propped up.

Take your time and shop around for the bed pillow that fits you best. Only you can know what's *just right*. Testing out a pillow in a store can be a challenge if there's no place to lie down with it. And store clerks can be less than knowledgeable about what they're selling. Consider your allergies first, because you won't want to buy one gigantic allergen for your room if down is what's filling your pillow. Synthetic and even hypoallergenic pillows are widely available now.

Tips to identifying a dead pillow:

1. When you take off the case and cover, are there old stains from sweat? If yes, it may not be dead yet, but it may smell pretty awful. If it passes the test but has smelly stains, I would get another one, anyway. Don't try to cover it up with perfumes or sprays, as these, too, can be allergens.

2. For natural pillows: If you fold over your pillow in half and it just lies there, you have a dead pillow. You can do this test with you arm, too. Just extend your arm out and hang the pillow across your arm; does it fold all the way over? That would be a dead pillow. If you have a king-size pillow, you will need to fold it in thirds, and if it does not spring

back, you have a problem. For synthetic pillows: Fold the pillow in half or thirds, depending on size, and add a ten-ounce weight on top (such as a sneaker). Then remove the weight. If the pillow releases back into shape, it's still good.

To recap: if every night you scrunch up your pillow and fold it in half like a neck-roll just to get it to fit comfortably underneath your head, you're in dire need of a new pillow. Certainly if your pillow is dirty, stained, torn, or if it smells bad, you also need a new bed pillow. Depending on the age for your bed pillow, over 50 percent of its weight is comprised of dead skin cells, mold, mildew, fungus, dust mites, and their lovely feces. (Makes you want to go get a new pillow today!)

Soft, medium, or firm pillows? The answer might depend on how you position yourself when you sleep. Generally speaking, side sleepers do best with thick, extra-firm pillows because they need to fill the space between their neck and shoulders to get correct alignment. Stomach sleepers like the softest pillows or no pillow at all because they do not need their head to be raised and can keep their spine aligned better with softer pillows. Back sleepers are better using a medium pillow.

Having said that, however, focus more on what feels good to you when you test your potential candidates out in the pillow shop. Don't worry so much about how the manufacturer or store categorizes the pillow; go with your own instinct. If you've got any physical ailments that can be relieved by a pillow, such as arthritis, position pillows to cushion your joints. Don't be afraid to consider body, back, and knee pillows if those provide more comfort to you.

Shopping for the perfect pillow is intimidating: Any single store will carry dozens of brands with their own labels and fancy names. Pillows come in all shapes, sizes, and fillers. Let's review the main filler options, which is the first decision you have to make.

Down. If you like a very soft pillow, there is no substitute for down. Allergy-free down is now created using a blend of super-clean pure down and milkweed clusters called syriaca that bind to the down plumes, helping the down's longevity and making it further allergy free. This type of down is often called hypodown, and while it can be expensive, it lasts a great deal longer than the cheaper grade down pillows. Interestingly, the reason a lot of people are allergic to down is because the manufacturers don't clean the down efficiently, so the dirt on the feather quills causes problems. The good down products are those that have gone through a rigorous cleaning process. The caveats to down:

- "Pure down" is a loose term. So is "all down." These pillows can also contain a lot of feathers or other fill. "Blended" down pillows are just that—a blend of both down and feathers. A "down around" pillow has a center chamber of down with feathers all around it.
- Goose down is softer and more expensive than duck down. And not all geese produce the same soft down.

Synthetic down and polyesters. There are lots of choices here, the most popular one being Primaloft. These are much cheaper than the hypoallergenic pure downs, but they won't last as long. The fibers used in polyester fills come in a variety of types: super slick, slick, blended, and dry fibers. General rule: The slicker the fiber, the more it moves as you move. In other words, the better the fiber, the slicker and more silky it will feel. Pillows begin to flatten when, over time, the air trapped inside the fiber gets exhausted.

Wool. Naturally hypoallergenic, wool pillows will resist dust mites and mold and will last a long time. They will wick away moisture and keep you cool in the summer and warm in the winter. But they can be on the firm side and not for someone who's got to have a sumptuously soft pillow. An alpaca-wool blend can be a good choice. Because alpaca wool is softer than cashmere, it provides a wool pillow's durability but is noticeably softer.

Cotton. Like wool, cotton is naturally hypoallergenic, resists dust mites and mold, and is a breathing fiber. Cotton pillows also tend to be on the firm side, so they're suitable for those who prefer flat pillows. Cotton pillows are best for people with multiple chemical sensitivities.

Latex. This is the firmest pillow of all. Natural latex resists dust mites and mold. Latex pillows are often contoured for neck support, and they maintain their shape for years. Perfect for those who need to align their back and neck. If you're the type who likes to scrunch your pillow behind your neck, however, this is not the pillow for you. These pillows also tend to be visually unappealing, disqualifying your bed from making the cover of a catalog. (Not that they aren't the optimal pillows for you, however!)

Memory Foam: How Does *That* Work?

The technology behind memory foam, short for visco-elastic memory foam, originates from NASA, which first developed this material in the 1970s to help astronauts during their launches into space. Because an astronaut's body has to absorb tremendous G-forces at blast-off, the idea was to create a material that could conform to an individual's shape and hold that conformity—even when the body moved or shifted position. What developed was this visco-elastic foam that responds to weight and temperature; it not only softens and molds itself to whatever shape is applied via weight, it also comes back to a normal shape once pressure is removed from the surface. It "resets" itself. This allows an even distribution of pressure or body weight over the entire surface of the foam, which can quickly adapt to any body movements.

Temperature-sensitive memory foam reduces pressure points by continuously molding and adjusting to the shape of your body as you move and shift your weight. Traditional cushioning materials, on the other hand, don't redistribute weight the way visco-elastic can, thus potentially creating and exacerbating pressure points. This is why it's said that visco foam is a true cushioning foam and not a support foam. Although experiments started in the 1980s to bring NASA's ideas over to the consumer market and perfect them for other uses, memory foams didn't reach the pillow and mattress world until Tempur-Pedic came out with a visco-elastic memory mattress in the early 1990s. Some have suggested that one tosses and turns 80 percent *less* when sleeping on visco foam.

Memory foam. Some people swear by these pillows. But a few caveats to consider are:

- They can emit an unpleasant, chemical odor.
- They can make you too hot, making you wake up at night in a sweat.

- Not all memory foam products are created equal. High-quality memory foam is the right size, has no fillers, is based on good chemistry, has good cell structure, has the right temperature sensitivity, as well as good response time.

They now make layered foam with different support levels and memory foam inserts that can be quite comfortable.

RUB-A-DUB-DUB: THE RULES TO WASHING AND DRYING

When? Wash entire pillows infrequently—once every two to three months (you can go longer depending on the type of pillow). Wash pillow covers frequently—once a month. If your pillows don't have a zip-off cover that can be washed, consider purchasing some (these are not the same as pillow*cases*). Using pillow covers will help your pillows last longer, shielding them from stains and moisture. In lieu of an actual cover, you can also use two pillowcases inverted.

How? Hand-wash polyester, foam, feather, and down pillows with a fabric soap in cool water or in a machine. Wash two at a time on a short, delicate cycle. Rinse thoroughly. You can machine dry all pillows— except foam—on low or no heat. Ring out pillows before drying. Read your labels for specifics. Add a couple of tennis balls to the dryer for feather and down pillows so they fluff up.

A pillow may last anywhere from twelve months to three years or longer. Yes, it's a huge range. Natural pillows last a little longer than synthetic pillows (five to seven years for a natural pillow, versus two to three for a synthetic). And you get what you pay for. Think how much you spend on other items you use every day, like clothes and accessories. Your pillow is used every night, for about 8 hours, which equals 2,920 hours per year. Don't underestimate the overall value of a good pillow. Spend wisely.

Pic-a-Pillow: A Step-by-Step Guide for Pillow Selection

1. **Feel, Touch, Squish, Test Out**

There's no better way to pick a pillow than to have your own set of criteria and go with your gut instinct. Remember the six elements to a pillow: 1) fill/

fiber, 2) fill weight, 3) quality of fill, 4) overall size, 5) fabric, and 6) chemistry. If you want to try matching your main sleeping position with your pillow type, here are the general guidelines (note the caveat below):

On-the-back sleepers *might* need a flatter pillow for head and neck alignment. It should be soft yet supportive. If you experience stiffness or neck pain with your current pillow, try something a bit more supportive.

On-the-side sleepers *might* need a firmer pillow, preferably one as thick as the distance between your ear and outside shoulder.

On-the-stomach sleepers *might* need a very soft pillow (or no pillow) for their head but may need one for under their stomach to avoid lower back pain.

Caveat: I used the word "might" in the guidelines above because there is no definitive rule on pillow picking. How many of us actually sleep in a static position all night long? Not many. So, in some regards, the advice that you should match your main sleeping position with your pillow type is marketing hype. If you get a pillow that fits and meets your personal "squish factor" standards, then it should work in *all* sleeping positions.

2. Filler Up!

Consider hypoallergenic or synthetic fills if pure down is a severe allergen for you or your bedmate. Blends with feathers and down are also available. Few people have issues with wool and cotton fills. Some people, especially those with neck pain, really enjoy the memory foam pillows. Quality memory foam, however, is based on quality chemistry behind it. Chemistry can also be a factor when it comes to choosing pillows with antimicrobial treatments, which you'll find in many synthetic fills. Keep in mind that to date there is no pillow-to-pillow comparison to tell us if one is better than another. It's a personal preference.

When it comes to "fill power," the higher the number, the higher the quality and the longer the life of the pillow. Top-of-the-line Hypodown pillows have a fill power of 800 and are supposed to last ten years (yeah, right!). Anything above 600 is a good fill power.

3. Size It Right

Make sure your pillows fit their covers and cases perfectly. Most people need only a standard-size pillow. Body pillows can be helpful for women who are pregnant, adding extra support under their bellies and in between the knees.

Try small pillows for in-between the knees.

You may also want to experiment with pillows uniquely shaped for maintaining position. For example, the hook-shaped Sleep Posture Pillow cradles you in a semifetal position that prevents you from wiggling (and disturbing your bed partner). Be mindful of marketing hype. Snore-reduction pillows have hit the market, but there's no such thing as an anti-snore pillow. What's more, specialty coverings/casings have made the covering or ticking on pillows not matter. One company (Carpenter) uses a material shown to increase oxygen levels in the blood for diabetics!

4. **Discern Decorative from Truly Functional**
   If you're into decorating your bed with fashionable, eye-catching pillow designs, be sure to remove them prior to sleeping. These are not usually supportive and will be too stiff.

DUVETS AND BLANKETS

Duvet covers have gained a lot of popularity, mainly because you can fill them with a luxurious soft comforter and have flexibility with using different covers throughout the year. Again, if you've got allergy issues with down, you can't go for the down comforter—even if it's covered up by the duvet.

Wool blankets can be problematic, too, if they'll cause itching and scratching. Today, there are so many synthetic blends available that mimic natural fibers that it pays to experiment with a few to find the ones that you like and that won't affect your ability to sleep well.

Also remember that you should change your blankets seasonally. Summer should be reserved for lighter materials and winter for heavier materials.

SAFETY FIRST

A restful night never happens if your bedroom doesn't make you feel safe. This may sound like a strange topic, but it's relevant—especially if you live alone and the onset of night makes you nervous, scared, or worried about intruders. Do everything in your power to ensure your safety. This may include having a house or door alarm, a dog, or using night-lights that make you feel extra safe.

MATTRESSES

Buying a mattress these days is like buying a car. Not only is the mattress market fiercely competitive, but stepping into a mattress superstore can feel like you're walking onto a dealership lot. With so many brands to choose from, how can you discern the good from the bad? Can you really find a good mattress at Costco or Wal-Mart that compares to mattress specialty shops? Adding to the confusion are those long advertisements and infomercials that talk about new and sometimes strange technology going on in the mattress-manufacturing business. One particularly comedic ad shows a kid jumping up and down on one side of the mattress while a glass full of red wine rests undisturbed on the other side.

If you're not a mattress expert, it's hard to tell one box of metal, foam, fuzz, and fabric from another. Sales pitches can be convincing, especially if you're not into putting as much time and research into buying a mattress as you would a car. Compounding the problem is the fact that model names differ from store to store, making it impossible to comparison shop. And prices vary so much that the $1,300 mattress set you look at one day can cost $2,600 the next.

Let me attempt to end the confusion right here by starting with this: I can't tell you which mattress is perfect for *you*. All but the cheapest mattresses are apt to be sturdy, but there are no reliability data for specific models or even brands. I repeat: *There is no data to suggest one brand over another—no matter what your sales guy says!* Retailers will say that no brand is less trouble prone than another. Industry-wide, less than 1 percent of mattresses are returned for warranty failures such as broken springs. And, as you can imagine, comfort is relative. So what we've got is a very subjective industry.

More people are going for the bigger beds now. Queen is the most widely sold size, and kings account for nearly 10 percent of the market. Mattresses aren't built like they used to be, either. Quality has risen across the board. Many are almost twice as thick as they were a decade ago—up to twenty inches—and they're also heavier. Most have cushioning on the top only, so manufacturers no longer suggest that you flip them. (It's still a good idea to rotate most from front to back to even out wear.) Among major brands, Serta continues to make some two-sided mattresses, each side equipped with individually controlled air chambers. Mattress makers are using more foam, including latex and visco-elastic memory foam, which, as I've already covered, make for body-hugging, longer-lasting padding. Having less polyester fiber helps prevent the mattress from packing down. Mattresses that absorb movement and prevent the transfer of motion, say, from one side of the bed to the other, are also popular these days. Both Tempur-Pedic and Simmons Beautyrest boast of these characteristics to their products.

Other improvements in the last decade include stain resistance. Serta's top-of-the-line Perfect Sleeper, for example, has stain-proof yarns; Simmons' stain-resistant HealthSmart mattress has a Teflon-coated, zippered top pad that is machine washable (so you're not sleeping in sweat, oil, and dust mites). This is really nice when you want the cleanest possible sleep surface. So-called Eurotops have gotten popular, too. These are separate layers of padding sewn tightly onto a mattress. Eurotops differ from older pillowtops, or cushy pads sewn loosely atop a mattress that are prone to sagging over time. One company, Kingsdown, has taken a decidedly scientific bent. They have you lie on their mattress (which is embedded with a pressure-sensor system) in the store and determine the appropriate firmness for both you and your bed partner. They can then custom make your bed based on your individual cushioning and support needs. (I was very impressed with their technology.)

With all these new features and innovations comes a higher price. Rising material costs also contribute to the equation as plush fabrics like fancy damask, jersey knit, microsuede, wool, cashmere, and even silk get incorporated.

I'll repeat this one more time before moving on: Selecting a mattress is a personal choice. Go with what your body tells you when you test out the different types and brands in stores. Don't judge a mattress by its name, celebrity endorsement, or by what the salesperson tells you. Use your gut instinct.

Consumer Reports receives more inquiries about mattresses than about any other product except cars.

Uncovering the Facts Beneath the Fiction in the Mattress Industry
(Adapted from *Consumer Reports,* June 2005)

Fact: Coil count is *not* critical. Any number above 390 in a queen-size mattress should be plenty.

Fiction: Firmer is better. This may be true for some people—but not everyone. The best bed is the one that's most comfortable to you.

Fact: A higher price does not guarantee a better bed. Anything but the cheapest mattress can be good. The best bed is the one you're comfortable sleeping in.

Fiction: Fancy fabrics like silk, cashmere, and wool make for a more comfy bed. These fabrics add more to the price than to the comfort level. When you cover your mattress with a pad and sheets, you can't directly feel the mattress's surface, anyway.

Fact: A mattress can outlive you to some degree. Changes in the human body tend to make a mattress less comfortable long before it wears out.

Fiction: You must include a box spring to save the warranty. Despite sales pressure to buy both mattress and foundation, it's not always required. You may be able to keep your old box spring if it's in good shape.

Fact: Warranties *will not* cover a sagging mattress if it's under certain specifications. Manufacturers say a mattress can compress by as much as one and a half inches before it's considered defective.

Fiction: All beds are equally fire-resistant. California has the strictest fire-safety codes, but your state may allow mattresses to be sold that are not up to the same high standard.

Fact: Salespeople receive financial incentives to sell certain brands and models. These incentives are called SPIFs (for "sales person incentive funds"), and commissions can amount to about $100 a bed.

The Step-by-Step Mini-Guide to Choosing a Mattress

1. Determine your need for a new mattress.

   How old is your current one? If more than seven years, it's probably time. Also consider a new mattress if you wake up tired or achy; if you sleep better at hotels than at home; if your mattress looks saggy or lumpy; or if you're over age forty and your mattress is five to seven years old. Bodies tolerate less pressure as they age.

2. Pick a size. Go bigger if your current bed feels too small. Get all the room you need.

3. Decide between innerspring, memory foam, and inflatable mattresses.

"Innerspring" mattresses are the more common choices; memory foam, on the other hand, is what you see advertised in specialty stores or on TV (discussed in detail on page 107). Developed to protect astronauts against G-forces, memory foam is heat-sensitive and conforms to your body (e.g., Tempur-Pedic). Not all memory foam feels the same, and it can take time to get used to. Just like the memory foam pillows, also be aware it can have a distinct (chemical) smell to it. Inflatable mattresses let you choose a different firmness for each half of the bed (e.g., Select Comfort). According to *Consumer Reports* magazine, one mattress does not perform better than another so it's all personal preference.

4. Check out your options in person. Avoid online, phone, and catalog shopping (unless you've already done your research in person).

Go for what mattress feels best for you, as there is no one-size-fits-all mattress. Don't go by name and price only. Spend a good fifteen minutes—on each potential candidate in the store—lying down on each side and on your back. Don't go on a Saturday afternoon. Visit a store late in the evening after a full day of work. Wear sweatpants and a loose shirt (similar to what you might wear to bed). Make sure to test each mattress out in as real a setting as possible.

5. Try and get a deal on the box spring, which is generally just a wood frame enclosing stiff wire and covered with fabric matching the mattress's. If your current box spring is only a few years old, with no serious wear and tear, consider using it with a new mattress. If the old box has bouncy springs instead of stiff wire, it needs to be replaced. Some salespeople will tell you that you'll violate the warranty if the mattress and box spring are not sold as a set. You should go to the manufacturer's Web site and get this type of information beforehand. Go to the source before you deal with the salespeople.

6. Check return and warranty policies. Some retailers allow you to

return a mattress within a certain time period, often with a fee. Note that warranties typically are hard to enforce. They don't usually cover normal wear and comfort.

7. Wait for sales (specialty mattresses, however, rarely go on sale).

8. Ask if you can get your old mattress picked up when the new one arrives. Make sure your sales agreement includes a no-substitutions clause so that if the bed you ordered is out of stock, you won't be surprised with another type. When it's delivered, look for damage, and request a replacement if necessary. If they bend it around a corner, it can cause significant damage to the wire frame. Make sure you get what you ordered; check the mattress name with the invoice.

> **Q.** It's made in Sweden, sells for a high, nonnegotiable price in boutique showrooms, and is backed by some pretty convincing advertisements. Is it worth it? Will it change my sleeping experience forever?
>
> **A.** A lot of specialty mattresses have hit the market in recent years—some of them touted by Hollywood celebrities. You don't always get what you pay for in the mattress department, however. In polls conducted on people who've purchased some of the priciest mattresses around, responses ran the gamut from yea to nay. This points to the subjectivity of mattress buying and the need to spend more time testing them out in stores than reading *Consumer Reports* and going on the advice of others. You wouldn't buy a car without test-driving it, and you shouldn't buy a mattress without taking the same precautions.

Smell

Your olfactory system (sense of smell) is one of the most influential sensory parts of the body. It's also one of the oldest and most vital components of the brain; scents stimulate your command center for emotion, motivation, and memory. Smell is also the only sense to travel directly to the cerebral cortex, where sensory perception occurs, rather than being relayed first through the thalamus. As such, it's considered the most primitive of the five senses. For most animals, it is the primary mode of communication and influences many important functions, including reproduction and taste. Let's not forget about how it can influence our sleep, too. An unfriendly odor wafting in the bedroom can greatly affect our ability to fall asleep. Have you ever stopped to consider the odors lingering in your bedroom?

Questions to ask yourself:

- What are the smells in your bedroom without anyone in it?
- What odors do you or your bed partner bring to it? Gas? Body odor? Perfume?
- Do you or your bedmate exercise before bed?
- Do you have air fresheners?
- Have you ever tried aromatherapy?
- Do you live in an older home with mold/mildew?
- Do you live near the water, especially the ocean?
- How close is your bedroom to your bathroom?

Be careful not to over-odorize your bedroom, but if smell is a problem, consider aromatherapy. Recent studies have offered evidence that aromatherapy can not only lift your spirits, but possibly reduce anxiety, agitation, and even pain—all good effects for inducing sleep. Specifically, consider relaxing smells such as lavender, rose, vanilla, and chamomile. Aromatherapy oils can be infused in the air, rubbed on the skin, or even ingested. Although powerful, these are great "mood setters." For safety reasons, never light aroma candles. Use sprays, powders, or even fresh flowers (if no one is allergic). Consider some of the current products to reduce or mask odors (e.g., Febreze). But remember those are simple, immediate solutions. Find the source of the odor. In addition, ask your bed partner to wear fresh bedclothes, not a T-shirt that he or she may have worn all day or the same underwear. This can help reduce body odor and set the stage for sleep by making putting on your "sleep clothes" a cue before bed.

Q. Can I actually smell during my sleep? I've seen products that claim to help me stay asleep with special scents. Is that true?

A. Smell is more of an issue at bedtime, when you're trying to fall asleep and reduce your anxiety level. Recent data suggests that you cannot smell while sleeping, so beware of advertisers who make you think you can smell their products while sleeping.

Taste

Eating too close to bedtime can be a major cause of insomnia and troubled sleep. Do you eat a snack before bed? How much time typically passes between your last meal and bedtime? Do you suffer from GERD (gastroesophageal reflux disease)?

If your digestive tract is trying to process food while you're trying to settle into a long and cozy slumber, your body might find it difficult to conduct these two competing tasks. Experiment with the timing of your meals and snacks before bedtime to see what works best. I tell my patients to avoid large meals within three hours of bedtime. And if they are going to have a small snack just beforehand, I suggest a complex carbohydrate with a little protein, plus calcium: such as a piece of whole wheat toast with a thin slice of low-fat cheese on top, or try a piece of plain cheesecake. The lactose intolerant can choose peanut butter as a topping, as long as they stay within 200 calories for the entire snack. I also remind them to be careful about any caffeinated foods and beverages close to bedtime.

Remember, what you eat—especially when lying down—can give you gas. This can be quite unpleasant for you and your bed partner.

> By combining an ample dose of carbohydrate together with a small amount of protein (which contains the amino acid tryptophan), your brain produces serotonin, which is known as "the calming hormone." You'll learn about the best bedtime snacks in a later chapter.

Attention GERD Sufferers:
How to Avoid That Burn at Night.

- Avoid lying down for two to three hours after eating. (Lying down can push stomach juices into your esophagus, causing heartburn.) Similarly, be careful when bending and lifting for the same reason.
- Avoid eating large meals and snacks just before bedtime.
- Avoid tight clothing over your stomach.

Raising the head of your bed six to eight inches can help those who suffer from acid reflux or from poor circulation in their legs. You can do this by putting blocks underneath your bed frame or by placing a foam wedge under the head of your mattress. Using extra pillows will not work.

Cramped Quarters

What do you do if you live in a matchbox New York City apartment? If you've got little room to play with and your kitchen sink lies a few feet away from your bed, turning your "bedroom" into a sanctuary for sleep can be tough. But not impossible. Follow these tips:

- Position your bed in a way that signifies it's part of its own entity or room (instead of being another piece of furniture in the main room). Consider the use of a room divider or a screen. If you sleep on a pull-out couch, pull it out two to three hours before you are ready to retire, thus setting the mood for sleep.
- Decorate the area around the bed differently from the rest of the apartment. It should visually stand out separately. Use cool, calming colors and textures (blues, greens, and purples).
- Splurge on good bedding materials that are comfortable for you.
- Keep high-wattage lights away from the "bedroom" setting. Install low-wattage lights anywhere near the bed or add dimmers to all the switches, and again set the mood for sleep two to three hours before you retire.
- Position your entertainment, television, and/or computer area so it's not directly aligned with your line of vision when you're in bed. Again, consider the use of covers for the monitor and turning off the CPU itself.
- If you can't paint the bedroom area (which is the case for many apartment dwellers unless you get specific permission from the landlord), evoke the same mood and feeling by your choice of colored draperies for the window (consider blackout shades), frames around wall hangings and photos, and linens on the bed.

- Face the bed west if possible so that you don't get direct sunlight in the morning.
- Use eye shades.

The Best and Worst Cities for Sleep

According to a study done by Sperling's BestPlaces, a research firm in Portland, Oregon, that specializes in studies ranking and rating United States metro areas, the top-ten metro areas for best sleep are:

1. Minneapolis–St. Paul, MN
2. Anaheim, CA
3. San Diego, CA
4. Raleigh–Durham–Chapel Hill, NC
5. Washington, D.C.
6. Bergen-Passaic, NJ
7. Chicago, IL
8. Boston, MA
9. Austin, TX
10. Kansas City, MO

And the ten most sleep challenged places are:

1. Detroit, MI
2. Cleveland, OH
3. Nashville, TN
4. Cincinnati, OH
5. New Orleans, LA
6. New York, NY
7. Las Vegas, NV
8. Miami, FL
9. San Francisco, CA
10. St. Louis, MO

The study also found that the single greatest factor identified by people who reported themselves as being happy (feeling healthy and full of energy) was having restful sleep. The purpose of the study was to identify where people are likely to have the easiest and most challenging time having restful sleep, and which factors in each city contribute to its ranking. For more on how this study was done and what factored into their ranking, go to www.bestplaces.net/docs/studies/AmbienSleep.aspx.

THE BEDROOM CHECKLIST

The following are the main topics covered in this chapter. Go through it once more with the vision of your bedroom in mind. It will help you know what to tackle first in modifying your current setting.

- furniture arrangement and special layout
- wall colors, paint, or paper
- wall hangings and adornments
- quality of mattress
- bedding linens
- pillows, blankets, covers
- source and intensity of light (natural and artificial, including monitors)
- source and intensity of sounds (natural and artificial, including TV)
- odors
- air quality
- temperature and humidity

SoundSleepSolutions.com

Don't forget to check out my Web site at www.soundsleepsolutions.com. There, you can write to me about your personal experiences with sleep, share your own tips on an active message board, and ask questions. I'll post the most frequently asked questions with their answers and possible solutions. Your questions will contribute to an online and active Troubleshooting Guide.

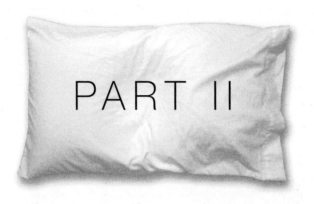

PART II

From Waistlines to
Face Lines:
You Are What You Sleep

CHAPTER 5

Snooze to Lose: Sleep and How It Affects Weight Loss . . . and How Sleep Is Cosmetic Medicine

If you've ever participated in a weight-loss program and had disappointing results, you may have been doing everything right except for getting a good night's rest. The vast majority of these programs never mention sleep's role in the whole equation. The same holds true for beauty products and "systems" that line department store shelves and infiltrate your television. Diets and skin care products are marketed brilliantly, and they all tend to be quite convincing. You read somewhere that "Results may vary" in fine print, but you never learn what factors can cause these variations.

Before you blame your poor results on bad genes or the program itself, stop and take a good look at your sleep habits. How fast are you chasing sleep while also in pursuit of losing weight or reversing the visible signs of age? Does sleep get left behind while you worry about everything else in life?

To accomplish either of these goals, you must consider a parallel commitment to getting more sleep. Otherwise, you can do all the sit-ups and calorie counting you want, or spend a fortune on designer beauty products, and still come out not looking or feeling any younger. I'm serious. If I could finish the "Results may vary" disclaimer, I'd add ". . . DE-PENDING ON SLEEP HABITS."

The first part of this book outlined some of the ways in which you can achieve a good night's sleep. Now it's time to learn what quality sleep will actually do for you physically—other than just make you feel great. Once you understand the significance of sleep to your health, you'll value it more and work toward getting it routinely no matter what.

You might have read the headlines or heard the news in recent years as the mainstream media began to report the buzz going on in sleep medicine. Fantastic new sleep research has uncovered new knowledge that is currently revolutionizing many industries, from the fitness and health to the diet, weight loss, cosmetic, and general medical. A stunning find came in late 2004, when researchers showed the strong connection between sleep and the ability to lose weight: The more you sleep, the better your body can regulate the chemicals that control hunger and appetite. Of course, as soon as everyone heard this news, they began to think twice about their sleep habits and the deprived lives they led when it came to sleep. It was good news for the field of sleep medicine, which gained greater recognition and a stronger foothold in general medicine. At the time the news hit, however, the National Sleep Foundation released its annual report that said three in four people frequently have sleep problems. That's almost the same number of overweight and obese people. I immediately wondered what could happen if instead of talking about just diet and exercise with regard to losing weight, we urged people to focus on sleep first, then diet and exercise?

If you tried one or two of the Action Plans detailed in the first part of this book and now you're getting through your days a little easier and with a bit more energy, that's a positive change in your life. Congrats. You may not realize it today, but just by learning how to get better, higher-quality sleep you've deposited more years into your bank of longevity.

As I'm about to show you in Chapters 6 and 7, sleep is a natural weight manager, it's a natural cosmetic medicine, it's a way to a better sex life, and it's an excellent method for staying motivated, fit, creative, stress-free, and pain-free. We're going to take a break from the questionnaires and Action Plans so we can delve into the details of what you can get out of a good night's rest.

Snooze to Lose

The average person has 40 billion fat cells. They multiply, they're almost impossible to kill, and you know what happens to them when the weight starts packing on. The truth about weight loss can be hard to accept: There is no secret. It's a mathematical equation: If the calories you consume are greater than the calories you burn, you'll gain weight. And if the calories you consume are *less* than the calories you burn, you'll *lose* weight. So if you want to find a secret somewhere in that equation, it's in boosting your burning capacity and limiting your consumption. And here's the kicker: Sleep can do just that.

Sleep and weight loss share a hidden, albeit powerful bond that is just beginning to be clearly understood. It pretty much boils down to raging hormones—even though you're not a teenager anymore.

THE HORMONES THAT CONTROL YOUR LIFE

There's nothing very simple about hormones and how they work in your body to keep you alive and well. I hold a great respect for endocrinologists who study this complex realm of medicine and make sense out of the highly intelligent and elaborate connections between biological molecules that play a role in everything you do. No discussion about sleep can exclude them.

Hormone regulation is like an intricate dance that takes place every second in your body, and goes far beyond the action of commonly known hormones, such as testosterone and estrogen, that control your reproductive system. In fact, from the moment of conception you are under the influence of a multitude of hormones, and this continues until death. If you flipped through an endocrinology medical textbook, you'd be amazed by how prevalent hormones are from head to toe. You would also be astounded at the number of pathways these "masters of ceremonies" partake. By the time you finish this sentence, millions of hormone pulses will have already taken place somewhere within you.

You can think of hormones as the messengers between various systems and command posts; they get produced in one part of the body, such as the thyroid, adrenal, or pituitary gland, pass into the bloodstream, and get carried to distant organs and tissues, where they act to modify structures and functions. Hormones act like traffic signs and signals—telling your body what to do and when, making sure its machinery runs smoothly and maintains equilibrium, or homeostasis. They are as much a part of your reproductive system as they are a part of your urinary, respiratory, cardiovascular, nervous, muscular, skeletal, immune, and digestive system. In short, they control just about every internal system. And lo and behold, their delicate balance relies on sleep.

Much of how you *feel*—tired, ravenous, full, excited, thirsty, hot, cold, stressed out—is due to hormones getting secreted and having an impact on your mind and body. Because your metabolism is the sum of all the chemical and physical changes that take place within your body, enabling its continued growth and function, your metabolism is at the mercy of these chemicals 24/7. Two hormones in particular tell you whether you're hungry or full, and whether or not you'd prefer the chocolate cake to cottage cheese. If you're wondering whether you can control any of these hormones so you'll start craving celery and be sickened by dessert, read on.

THE FIGHT FOR SATISFACTION BETWEEN GHRELIN AND LEPTIN

The two digestive hormones that hold the remote control to your feelings of hunger and appetite are ghrelin and leptin. As with many hormones, these two are paired together but have opposing functions. One gives the green light that says Go and the other emits the red light that says Stop. Ghrelin (your "Go" hormone) gets secreted by the stomach when it's empty and increases your appetite. It sends a message to your brain that says, "I'm hungry. Feed me." When your stomach is full, the other hormone—leptin—sends your brain the message that says, "Stop eating. I'm done." You can thank your fat cells for sending leptin out, allowing you to push away from the table. So how do these hormones tie in to sleep?

Inadequate sleep creates an imbalance of both ghrelin and leptin. One study at the University of Chicago in 2004 showed that when people were allowed just four hours of sleep a night for two nights, they suffered a 20 percent drop in leptin and an increase in ghrelin. These sleep-deprived participants had a 24 percent increase in hunger and a 23 percent increase in appetite. *Hunger* is the feeling of wanting to eat and your *appetite* is the physical need to eat until full. (Think of hunger as the sensation that precedes eating.) If your brain isn't getting the message that you are full, you keep eating and eating and eating.

Fact: Ever wonder if some people have totally defunct appetite and satiety hormones? Prader-Willi syndrome (PWS) is a complex genetic disorder in which people experience a chronic feeling of hunger that often leads to excessive eating and life-threatening obesity. Because of a dysfunction in their hypothalamus, which usually sends out the messages, their brain never gets clued in to that feeling of fullness. Their urge to eat is physiological and overwhelming, and there is no cure. PWS, while rare, is the most common genetic cause of obesity; it's difficult to control and requires constant vigilance. Those with PWS typically have serious sleep disorders and are urged to undergo sleep studies to help alleviate respiratory problems that can be fatal.

Sleep loss, in a sense, disconnects your brain from your stomach. Have you heard of "mindless eating"? Not only is the act of eating unconscious, but you also have a hard time controlling *what* you eat. The Chicago study also found that participants' appetite for calorie-dense, high-carbohydrate foods like sweets, salty snacks, and starchy foods increased by 33 to 45 percent when they only slept four hours a night. This translates to two strikes against you: Sleep loss deceives your body into believing it's hungry (when it's not), and it also tricks you into craving foods that can sabotage a healthy diet. You'll want the cake and ice cream instead of the bowl of fruit and yogurt. And you won't be able to stop eating as easily.

This study was not a fluke. Other prestigious institutions have generated similar results, proving that ghrelin and leptin are, indeed, strongly influenced by sleep. How many hours do you need exactly to keep these hormones in balance? Eight or nine? At least five? I wish I could give you a clear-cut answer. As I've already explained, everyone has a different sleep number. So it depends on your individual body's needs. The overall response to these hormones may be more individual than we think. Your environment, dietary habits, exercise patterns, personal stress levels, and especially your genetics may all influence the production of leptin and ghrelin, as well as your response to them.

HFCS *NOT* TO THE RESCUE

One of the worst ingredients lining our supermarket shelves and ruining our quest for weight loss is HFCS—or high fructose corn syrup. Go ahead and take a look in your kitchen cupboards and refrigerators. See how many times you find this listed in the ingredients on labels. Cereals. Sodas. Salad dressings. Condiments (ketchup). Ice cream. Focus on processed and sweetened foods. Don't forget to check out anything specifically labeled "fat free," "lite," or "low fat." Even if you typically buy all-natural, organic foods, I bet you'll find some HFCS lurking somewhere.

Surprised? I wouldn't normally mention HFCS with regard to sleep, but it relates directly to ghrelin and leptin, which we've already seen connect to sleep. Lack of sleep and HFCS both antagonize your weight-loss efforts—and they happen to be each other's accomplice! I'll explain how.

When food manufacturers want a product to taste even better, they will often resort to this highly processed sugar that offers no nutritional value whatsoever, as if they're trying to "rescue" a mediocre-tasting food and elevate its consumption worthiness. In doing so, they will actually take out a nutrient and substitute it with HFCS. A lot of "fat-free" products are made this way. They take out the fat, which can be good for you in a balanced diet (not to mention help you feel full sooner), and inject a type of sugar that is always bad for you. Fructose, the main ingredient in HFCS, is now being blamed for the rise in obesity as studies point to a link between a rapid rise in obesity and this cheap corn product used to sweeten soft drinks and food since the 1970s. Between 1970 and 1990, HFCS consumption increased by more than 1,000 percent, largely because the nation's soft drink manufacturers switched from sucrose to HFCS. HFCS packs more calories into food and beverages than most people realize. We're eating between 200 and 300 more calories per capita per day than we were three decades ago; and between one-third and one-half of those calories come from soft drinks.

What is "fructose" and how does it relate to sleep? First, fructose is not the same as the major component found in regular white table sugar, or glucose, which is the main source of fuel for the body and especially the brain. Second, unlike glucose, fructose doesn't trigger responses in hormones that regulate energy use and appetite. Fructose is more likely to be converted into fat. And it doesn't help keep your ghrelin and leptin hormones in check. HFCS inhibits leptin secretion, so you never get the message that you're full. Likewise, it never shuts off ghrelin, so, even though you have food in your stomach, you constantly get the message that you're hungry. Let's make the connections:

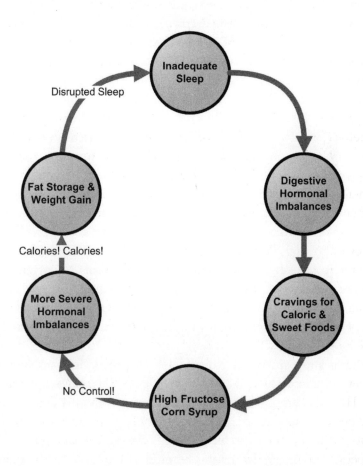

It's an ugly, vicious cycle that must be broken. You have to snooze to lose *and* lose to snooze, or you'll be caught in this fattening and sleepless cycle! Weight gain leads back to sleep loss because the more extra pounds you carry around, the harder it is to rest comfortably and avoid disrupted sleep. High fructose corn syrup, then, is a third party to obesity and sleep deprivation. And, unfortunately, it's snuck into the vast majority of our good-tasting food today.

BURN, BABY, BURN!

Although the jury is still out on exactly why this happens, sleep loss appears to interfere with the metabolism of carbohydrates, which, in turn, leads to more fat storage and a propensity to become overweight, if not outright obese. When sleep deprived, your body's ability to use glucose for energy drops about 30 percent. And when the body cannot use glucose effectively, it stays in the blood and increases your risk for type-2 diabetes. Even one week of sleep deprivation can cause a temporary diabetic effect! How scary is that? Of course, the sugar can't linger in the blood forever. Such an elevated blood sugar level promotes the overproduction of insulin—also a hormone—which then tucks away that unused energy in the form of fat. What's more, every time your body overproduces insulin, you become susceptible to so-called insulin resistance, at which point you can develop diabetes and no longer metabolize carbohydrates correctly. By then, your attempts to stay lean and healthy are all the more difficult.

A lot of popular diets do consider the insulin surge related to high-carbohydrate intake. The science behind the Atkins Nutritional Approach, Sugar Busters!, the Zone Diet, and low-carb diets in general, for example, is based on how your body responds to certain types of carbohydrates that either lead to burning the fuel for energy or, more likely, increasing fat storages.

Another key hormone in your body's fat-to-muscle ratio is growth hormone, or simply GH. As its name implies, GH plays a significant role in the maturation of a human being, but it's not only about getting Little Suzie all grown up. GH is very much a part of your adult life as well, acting similar to a conductor who orchestrates many functions at once. We'll be visiting this master hormone a bit later on in this chapter, but for now, understand that GH is a powerful anti-obesity hormone that decreases the rate at which your cells utilize carbohydrates and increases the rate at which they use fats (all good for weight loss). As soon as you hit deep sleep, about thirty to forty minutes after you first close your eyes, and then several more times throughout the night in your sleep cycle, your pituitary gland releases high levels of GH—the most it's going to secrete in twenty-four hours. So without that sleep, your levels of GH become significantly reduced, negatively affecting your proportions of fat to muscle. Over time, low GH levels are associated with high fat and low lean muscle.

> **Sleep Stat:** The more sleep deprived you are, the more likely you are to become obese. A study conducted with Columbia University's Mailman School of Public Health and the Obesity Research Center found that people between the ages of thirty-two and fifty-nine who sleep four hours or less per night are 73 percent more likely to be obese than those who sleep between seven and nine hours per night. Those who get five hours of sleep a night are 50 percent more likely to be obese than those who get seven to nine hours. And those who get six hours per night are 23 percent more likely to be obese. In which category do you fall?

MORE HORMONE ACTION

Two more hormones I want you to know about are cortisol and serotonin, both of which are linked to sleep and weight gain, but one is an enemy when it comes to any attempts at weight loss while the other is your friend.

You may already be aware that cortisol is a hormone related to stress. Whenever your body senses stress, this powerful biochemical gets released and, unfortunately, tells your body many things. But two things that are important for this discussion are that cortisol can tell your body to: 1) increase your appetite, and 2) stock up on more fat. So the next time you're stuck in endless traffic and worrying about picking the kids up on time or getting to your next appointment, consider what's going on at the cellular level: Your brain cells are sending "time to eat" messages, and your fat cells are being told to store as much fat as they can and hold on to that fat tightly.

Sounds counterproductive to what you'd like to have happen, but that's how your body naturally responds to stress. It automatically goes into a protectionist, survival mode, preserving itself by collecting and saving fat. You see, cortisol is your primary *catabolic* hormone, meaning it halts growth and reduces cellular synthesis (as opposed to increasing cell production and metabolism), causes muscles to break down, and assembles fat. As you might guess, you want to control your levels of cortisol; it's your nemesis for weight loss. But you can't do that well without enough sleep. Lack of sleep increases cortisol, resulting in your body storing fat, burning muscle—and *making you hungry by increasing your appetite*! In other words, it does the exact opposite of what you are trying to accomplish. And it's a quadruple whammy: High levels of cortisol also decrease your testosterone levels, which need to be high in order to keep your fat-burning–muscle-gaining processes going at full speed. Not surprisingly, cortisol levels are highest early in the morning and during periods of high stress, and lowest in early stages of deep sleep. (Some "fat-burning supplements" allege they can combat the effects of cortisol, but I challenge you to discover that a good night's sleep is the better, more effective remedy. As you'll learn in Chapter 11, you have to watch out for diet supplements that contain stimulants, which will hinder sound sleep and can ultimately work against your weight-loss goals.)

Serotonin, on the other hand, is your pleasure hormone . . . and your friend. Its strong connection to mood and emotion is why drugs to treat depression help increase the accessibility of serotonin levels in the brain. Inadequate sleep translates to less of this critical hormone getting released in the brain, and to compensate, you'll easily gravitate to foods with sugar (hence, "comfort foods") without even knowing it. And you know what that can mean for a waistline, much less a mood.

THE PRACTICAL VIEW

Insulin, leptin, ghrelin, GH, cortisol, serotonin—your head may be spinning in trying to remember these hormones and their exact functions. (Leave most of it to the endocrinologists.) While all this science is quite convincing, there is a practical point I want to make, too. Many patients report back to me that better sleep habits equate to more energy, which keeps them from relying on sweet foods and high-carb snacks to stay awake and feeling good. That alone automatically correlates to eating fewer calories, and having the energy to be active. Hormones and hardcore research aside, it doesn't take much to understand that the chance of succumbing to late-night cravings increases exponentially for every late hour of the day you stay awake. You've experienced this reality probably more than you'd like to admit. That's okay. Blame it on your hormones, but let's see if we can't help control those hormones with a slight shift in the way you spend your nighttime hours, a key part of my 28-night program. I guarantee you'll begin to see and feel a difference.

Let's sum this up here:

$$\textbf{Sleep Loss (Sleep Deprivation)} =$$
$$\uparrow \textbf{Appetite} + \downarrow \textbf{Metabolism} = \uparrow \textbf{Fat Storage}$$

It's as simple as that.

A TRUE STORY

Connie's story is one that many can relate to:

Connie W., forty-five, suffered from chronic lower back pain from an injury she received at age eighteen in a car accident. She also had a problem with insomnia, waking every couple of hours during the night and worrying about tasks—her To Do list—she hadn't accomplished. A single mother with two children under ten, Connie's weight began spiraling out of control soon after her divorce. She had tried several diet plans and even bought an exercise bike to motivate her to get active. But her results were always marginal at best. She repeatedly thought, No problem, just cut out a few extra snacks, exercise, and the weight will just drop off. Well, it just did not seem to work that way. Listen to her words:

> My doctor once again reminded me, "You know, if you could just lose a few pounds, most of your problems would go away." He said I wasn't twenty anymore, and that I needed to get my blood pressure and cholesterol levels under control or I'd need medication. I was slowing down on my food intake and taking the stairs instead of the elevator at work. Two weeks later, the scale wasn't going down. In fact, it went up! I had heard that muscle weighs more than fat, so I assumed I was replacing fat with muscle (yeah, right). The next week I had salads for lunch, skipped desserts, and reenacted my old gym membership. Back to the scale, but nothing had changed.
>
> I then decided to get serious. I went to my local bookstore and bought the latest top-selling "diet book" that had someone famous on the front cover. I also picked up another book to help count calories and carbohydrates. After following the books' instructions for two weeks, I got on the scale and noticed I weighed one pound less. I was very disappointed. What am I doing wrong? I

asked myself. Are those testimonials on the diet book real? I called my friend who has lost twelve pounds and I asked, "Okay, what is the big secret?"

As I sat drinking a diet drink she told me what to do, and I realized I was doing everything she told me. The only tip she offered that I hadn't tried yet was a food diary. I hung up the phone, felt depressed, and ate half a gallon of ice cream.

This is one of the most common stories I hear every day from both women and men. When Connie came to me, she was embarrassed and frustrated about her weight problem. At five feet four inches, she weighed 183 pounds and said she felt tired during the day, including the days when she believed she'd gotten a decent night's sleep. As a last-ditch effort, she had actually contemplated picking up smoking again—a habit she had broken ten years previously—in the hopes that it would help her lose weight. Her story continues:

I had tried everything in the books to lose weight. My back hurt constantly, so much that I could not sit through a movie. When I considered going in and seeing Dr. Breus for an official exam, I figured, okay, what do I have to lose? Nothing but the weight and pain. He made me do a sleep diary (not a food diary), and it showed exactly where I was going wrong when it came to getting quality sleep. I had never thought much about my daytime habits, which were clearly affecting my ability to get a good night's sleep. First, we had to figure out how many hours my body needed to feel awake and energetic all day long. Then he wrote out bedtime and morning routines that I was to practice religiously. We also took a good look at the medications I was downing for back pain and the tension headaches I got a few days a week.

It only took two weeks for me to see results. My diet and exercise program started to work, and believe me, it was no coincidence. I had tried this same program before and it had done little. Dr. Breus also gave me clear instructions for dealing with the insomnia and learning how to pay special attention to those days when it would be hard to follow a normal routine. I eventually lost more than thirty pounds. Best of all, my lower back pain nearly vanished. My headaches went away. Yesterday, my seven-year-old said, "Mommy, you're so pretty. You smile a lot now. I like it when you smile a lot."

For years I've been a witness, from a clinical standpoint, to sleep's profound role in the body. When the studies explaining the underlying science hit the major newswires in late 2004, I breathed a sigh of relief. I said, "Finally, more people will acknowledge sleep!"

The link between weight loss and sleep is so strong that I've had patients who clean up their sleep habits but still cannot lose weight. The problem? The *husband* keeps them up at night with his snoring, or thrashing around in the bed. So if your spouse is preventing you from getting quality sleep, you might as well be the one with the problem and you won't see acceptable weight loss from any diet program. Your focus, then, should be on finding the best way to become compatible sleep partners. This entails working with your partner as a team and figuring out the problem areas that you can solve together. Combined with your own diet and exercise habits, you can formulate a personal regimen that leads to results. The hardest part to your next diet is not going to be the diet—following what to eat and when—but, rather, focusing on your sleep and making sure you get enough quality Zs.

Bottom line: Make sleep your #1 priority when you embark on a diet and exercise program to lose weight and keep it off.

THE BRAIN'S LINK TO OVEREATING, OBESITY, AND INSOMNIA

Before moving on to the facts behind sleep as cosmetic medicine, I want to share another study that surfaced soon after the news about sleep's link to digestive hormones came out.

Stat: Nationwide surveys routinely find that more than 75 percent of women between the ages of twenty-five and fifty-four make diet resolutions each year or most years. Unfortunately, nearly 90 percent of those dieters often report either occasional or no success, with almost half losing little weight or actually gaining weight instead. A survey released in January 2006 revealed that roughly half of Americans (both men and women) make New Year's resolutions every year, but only about 11 percent of that half who make resolutions resolve to get more sleep. This poll also confirmed that the most common resolution is for the benefit of one's physical fitness (i.e., exercising more, losing weight, and having a healthier diet).

In April 2005, researchers at Yale University School of Medicine reported that there's a possible link between lack of sleep and obesity. The link has been traced to certain cells in the hypothalamus region of the brain (the region of the brain that contains several important centers controlling body temperature, thirst, hunger, eating, water balance, and sexual function) that are easily excited and sensitive to stress.

In a nutshell, when environmental or mental stress in daily situations overactivates these neurons, they may support sustained wakefulness, triggering sleeplessness and leading to overeating. So the more stress you have, the lower the threshold becomes for exciting these specific neurons. These neurons (which, for those who want to know, are called hypocretin/orexin cells) have a role in controlling arousal and alertness, two elements vital to survival. And their overactivation translates to more sleepless nights and the associated metabolic consequences (i.e., hormonal imbalances).

The take-home lesson from this study is to factor in the impact of stress. If you're looking to sleep better and manage weight effectively, your efforts will be aided enormously if you work on lessening the stress in your life. In the 28-night program, you'll learn a few meditation and relaxation techniques that will help you wind down prior to bedtime and lower your overall stress load. You can use these techniques any time of day so you can manage stress around the clock.

How Sleep Is Cosmetic Medicine

Improving your sleep habits to lose weight has an added bonus: You get to look better in terms of your skin, eyes, and even your hair. Imagine getting a free face-lift every night without surgery, and seeing a vast improvement in your complexion within forty-eight hours without the use of lotions, potions, and questionable pills. The cosmetic industry spends billions of dollars a year on marketing campaigns, and not one of them mentions how a good night's rest can help improve your beauty—or how their products can work better in combination with sleep.

You know that the appearance of your skin, eyes, and complexion reflects your age and health. You also know from experience that these features are compromised by sleep loss, especially if your debt is ongoing.

But do you know what goes on at the cellular level to cause these consequences, or how quality sleep can reclaim youthful beauty? I call sleep "cosmetic medicine" because it truly acts as an all-natural anti-aging solution (when used correctly, just like any other medicine). Here's why.

ENTERING THE REPAIR SHOP

Your body enters its maintenance and repair center while you sleep, or, as you're about to see, its own private "operating room." This is why dermatologists often suggest using your most "active" skin creams before bed. The body and its command center—the brain—are pretty efficient about knowing where and when to function maximally. While you sleep, your brain uses important neuronal connections that might otherwise deteriorate from lack of activity. During deep sleep, brain activity that control emotions, decision-making processes, and social interaction slows down. This allows you to maintain optimal emotional and social functioning when you are awake, when you'd need to use these functions. Your body can focus on other endeavors when it's asleep, and at the top of its list of priorities at night is cell growth and repair.

YOUR OWN PRIVATE OPERATING ROOM

Imagine that you're hiking on a trail through some tough elements—rain, rocks, mud, and lots of brush and trees. You get a cut on your leg, and then your shoelaces loosen. How hard would it be to continue walking and attempt to tend to your cut and shoelaces at the same time? Pretty hard. My guess is it would take a long time for the bleeding to stop and you would risk injuring yourself further. It would be nearly impossible to retie your laces while even moving at a slower pace. Now think of making a brief stop to care for the cut and retie your laces snugly. You get back to hiking quickly, your cut begins the healing process, and you probably hike stronger. The same scenario applies to sleep. During the day you expose your body to a host of elements, such as stress and UV rays, all of which contribute to the aging process. These are the rocks and brush your body endures day in and day out on its own "life trail." Sleep is the time-out your body requires to make necessary cellular repairs and zone in on restoring itself from the inside out. Deep sleep in particular becomes your own private operating room for all those nips and tucks that should naturally occur from within you. This is when your skin repairs itself, grows new cells, and fortifies its defenses against moisture loss and free radical damage (those loose cannons in the body that accelerate aging and can cause disease). Many cells also increase production of proteins (while decreasing breakdown) during this time, which in turn become the building blocks needed for cell growth and for repair of damage. And this is exactly why deep sleep may truly be "beauty sleep."

> Deep sleep refers to non-REM stages 3 and 4 in your sleep cycle. You reach deep sleep about thirty to forty minutes after you first close your eyes. Your brain waves become slow frequency and high voltage, and this slow-wave sleep is what's necessary for restoring your body. Deep sleep is famous for its growth-inducing properties, and plays a major role in maintaining your general health. It's difficult to rouse someone in deep sleep; it's as close to hibernating as one can get. (More on sleep cycles later in the book.)

Because millions of people cannot reach deep sleep on a regular basis, they lose out on visiting this grand operating room, which can explain why looking and feeling younger may seem like an uphill battle. They also lose out on getting special treatment from a highly qualified and talented doctor who does a lot of the miraculous work in this operating room. His name is Dr. GH.

I started to explain growth hormone earlier, telling how it affects the body's use of fats. Its function in the body is not isolated to metabolism, however. Released especially during deep sleep, GH has enormous rejuvenating effects that are all-encompassing, acting on both the mind and body. A protein that stimulates cells to increase in size and more rapidly divide, GH enhances the movement of amino acids through the cell membranes and increases the rate of protein synthesis. It's the primary hormone responsible for stimulating tissue repair, cell replacement, brain function, and enzyme production. GH affects almost every cell in the body, renewing the skin and bones, regenerating the heart, liver, lungs, and kidneys, bringing back organ and tissue function to more youthful levels. GH also revitalizes the immune system, lowers the risk factors of heart attack and stroke, improves oxygen uptake, and even helps prevent osteoporosis. For many, it acts like a natural cosmetic, restoring skin elasticity, smoothing wrinkles, and tending to hair and nails. If it sounds like the ultimate antidote to aging, or the body's natural wonder drug, it is. But the catch is, this antidote cannot be magically conjured up without adequate sleep. This doctor won't enter your operating room unless you reach deep sleep and stay there long enough without disruptions. I repeat: No deep sleep, no Dr. GH.

THE TRUTH ABOUT AGING

Like weight gain and the unrelenting equation of calories in versus calories out, there's an equation to aging that's hard to accept but is very true:

lifestyle + diet + genetics + fitness level + age + stress level + environment + other personal habits (including sleep) = how old you truly look and feel

Although we haven't figured out scientifically exactly the root causes of aging, we do know enough about age-related diseases to clue us in to the aging process and any attempts to slow it down or stop it. There's one type of aging in particular, however, that might surprise you and that is literally at the heart of the process. It's called arterial aging, and it refers to the inevitable decline of your heart and blood vessels through the years. And here's a most remarkable fact we cannot seem to fully explain: If you get less sleep than you need, you increase your arterial aging. This not only renders you at an increased risk for a heart attack, but it has a direct relationship to your appearance—how your skin looks and feels. Of course, arterial aging can also be accelerated by other variables, such as smoking, drinking, and obesity, but the link between sleep and arterial aging is stunning enough to pay attention to it.

PUTTING THE AIRBRUSH OVER WRINKLES

Your skin is a complex network of collagen and elastin fibers that work like rubber bands to keep your skin tight and young looking. As you know, long-term exposure to the sun has a nonreversible, damaging impact on your skin, accelerating its aging process by breaking down its natural fibers. Arterial aging has the same effect, destroying the elastin and eventually causing wrinkles. How so? As your arteries get older, they lose the capacity to nourish those skin fibers as well. As these fibers break down, they *stre-e-etch* out, causing scarring of the tissue. This leads the babylike skin to retract and form . . . voilà, wrinkles!

In addition, as your skin dries throughout the day, skin that's full of moisture will deflate and that stretched skin will fall into wrinkles. As you sleep, one of the ways your body lowers its temperature is by sweating. This helps moisture get back into the top layers of the skin, and fill the cells. When you use a nighttime moisturizer it also fills the skin's cells and makes it look full, much like adding water to a balloon—it gets round, full, and firm.

> One of the best things about sleep for your skin is that while sleeping, you are out of the sun (no damaging UV rays in bed), and your body can channel its nutrients to repairing your skin.

> **Warning:** Beware of some topical beauty products that guarantee to take years off your face. Smothering products over your face that claim to hydrate, build collagen, fill fine lines and wrinkles, etc., does not necessarily mean they get incorporated into your skin at the *cellular* level. They may improve the *appearance* of your skin by keeping the water in the cells, but, for the most part, YOU have to eat and hydrate well, nourishing your body from the inside out to take years off your face. There's no better setting than sleep for your body to use its own nutrients and collagen-building capacities on the inside.

Other than keeping arterial aging at bay and delaying the onset of wrinkles, can sleep do anything on a short-term basis, such as smooth out a complexion or tone down existing wrinkles overnight? You should already know the answers to these questions. Remember: Sleep provides the perfect operating room setting for conducting much-needed repair work. Yes, sleep is your personal airbrush. The overnight skin repairing that takes place is perhaps your greatest all-natural weapon against aging and the onset of wrinkles.

OPERATION SKIN, FACE, EYES, AND HAIR

Now, let's get to the details of those unwanted effects of sleep loss, especially the ones you can remedy with sleep:

Under-eye baggage. Awakening to puffy, swollen eyes is frustrating, especially when you know there's no simple ten-minute solution that will get you out the door looking brand new. Puffiness or bags under the eyes can be caused by several factors: fluid retention, irritation causing inflammation, loss of skin firmness and elasticity as we age, allergies, eye disorders secondary to medical disorders, fat deposits, and fatigue. Several of these triggers come from poor sleep.

Excess fluid (edema) under the eye is one of the major causes of eye "puffiness," and an increase in blood pressure is the likely culprit for many as a direct consequence of sleep deprivation. An elevated blood pressure causes vessels to constrict and invite fluid retention. Many of the known sleep disorders can also cause excess fluid or edema to occur not only in the eye area but in several parts of the body.

Is it possible for a person with retained fluid to reduce that baggage and puffiness under the eyes by getting a good night's sleep over time? Certainly. And if you can reduce the fluid retention, you'll also change the surrounding tissues for the better, especially since the accumulated excess fluid in the under-eye area may cause additional inflammation and swelling.

**Sleep Loss (Sleep Deprivation) = ↑ Blood Pressure +
↑ Fluid Retention = ↑ Puffiness and additional swelling
and inflammation**

Keep in mind that it's normal to have fat around the eye; the fat deposits are there to protect your eyes from injury. Your genes dictate much of how your eyes appear and age. The older you get, the easier it is for the tissues surrounding this fat to relax, and then the fat starts to stick out. Medical conditions can also change the appearance of the eye area, particularly thyroid problems like hypothyroidism (which can also be linked to sleep apnea). For most, however, getting enough sleep is all that's necessary. Avoiding excess alcohol will also alleviate eye bags (as well as disrupted sleep!).

Attention allergy sufferers: Those of you with allergies typically have issues with puffy, inflamed eyes. You also face the challenge of getting quality sleep when bothered by allergies during the night. Sometimes taking antihistamines can help reduce "baggy" eyes, but this can come with a hefty price tag because these medications can cause daytime sleepiness. What's worse, the act of coughing and sneezing itself can cause forced air to escape through the sinuses. This, in turn, pushes air behind the fat pockets under the eyes, which then causes those fat pockets to protrude forward. Ask your doctor how best to manage your allergies so that neither they nor your medication interfere with sleep.

Dark circles. Dark rings around the eyes—raccoon eyes—are typically blamed on poor sleep. But genetics bear a lot of the responsibility. The eyelid skin is the thinnest skin found anywhere in the body, so thin that it's almost transparent. The darkness under the eye is really circulating blood in the soft tissues beneath the skin, and your genes dictate the appearance of your under-eye area. However, because lack of sleep affects blood circulation, it's been theorized that sleep loss causes blood to pool under your eyes, thus adding insult to those dreaded dark circles. You can try to reverse this abnormal circulation by getting the right amount of sleep.

**Sleep Loss (Sleep Deprivation) =
↓ Circulating Blood in Soft Tissues + Delicate Skin Around Eyes =
↑ Dark Circles and Raccoon Appearance**

Red eyes. Red eyes simply mean you haven't rested them closed lately. When your lids are open (working very hard at watching, reading, absorbing a computer screen), your eyes are prone to dryness and irritation. You need shut-eye to keep the red out. At least five hours of sleep helps retinal membranes by allowing them to recharge from a long day of seeing. Allergies also can cause red eyes, but when your eyes are closed during sleep, it's pretty hard for allergens to irritate them. As you get sleepy, you blink more slowly. This can cause the eyes to dry and become itchy and red. Smoking will irritate the eyes, as will dry air.

Lifeless skin color. Proper circulation in your facial skin gives your face color. Rosy cheeks after being out in the cold, after you exercise, or even after feeling deep embarrassment, are the direct result of facial blood circulation. Sleep deprivation lowers circulation, which is why you lose facial color and look pale and washed out from poor sleep. You can't wake up glowing after only a few restless hours of Zs. Your cheeks should get "rosy" just before sleep, as this area helps cool blood to prepare your body for sleep.

Unhealthy hair. The connection between sleep deprivation and hair loss, breakage, damage, or growth is still a little fuzzy. Genetics do play a role in the quality and thickness of your head of hair, but environmental factors—including sleep—can play an even greater role. First, sleep deprivation causes a decrease in blood circulation, and blood circulation is how hair follicles gain nutrients, vitamins, and minerals. If your hair gets less food, it weakens and has difficulty growing. Second, animals studies show that severe sleep deprivation causes animals to shed hair. Third, sleep deprivation increases the body's level of stress, and increased stress can cause hair loss (and, don't forget, weight gain). Finally, here's the best evidence of all: Look at someone's hair who you know is sleep deprived. If she is not blessed with great hair to begin with, you'll likely notice that she's got thinning hair that appears difficult to manage.

Logging eight hours of sleep per night can make your "physical age" be as much as three years younger.

Shannon L.'s experience illustrates what a few minor changes in your sleep habits can do immediately to your appearance.

So I was feeling exhausted. I could not tell if it was work, my endless attempts at dating, or a mild case of depression. Either way, I was just plain tired. I was traveling for work constantly and I just never felt right. I contacted Dr. Breus and we discussed my sleep habits because I knew I was not getting enough sleep. I started a sleep diary and I learned how several of my sleep habits were not as good as I'd once thought. Together, we decided I should make some changes and see what happened.

It was hard for me to pinpoint when the change occurred, but it came soon after getting more quality rest. My dating life suddenly took off. I don't know if it was because I had more energy and guys were attracted to that, or if it was because I no longer had dark circles under my eyes. (I think I had gotten "used to" looking awful in the morning and later in the day, when the exhaustion set in.) All of a sudden I was finding myself getting compliments from men and feeling great. The most telling compliment came from an ex-boyfriend I bumped into at a bar one night. He said, "Wow, you look great. What did you do?" And when I thought about his question, I realized there was nothing different about me except that I was finally getting a reasonable amount of sleep. I told him, "I'm getting a good night's sleep; it's the new extreme makeover!" My mother also asked what my secret was. She said the change in my face was remarkable—my skin looked luminescent, radiating healthfulness. I wasn't even making any efforts with makeup, either. Of course, she wanted to know what product I was using or what diet I was on, and I told her it was simply a new sleep regimen. She didn't believe me!

CHAPTER 6

Sleep: The Medicine Necessary for Good Sex, and a Powerful Co-Partner with Exercise

Are you too sleepy for sex and exercise? Isn't the old "I have a headache" excuse the code phrase for "I'm too tired"? And when you're looking for an excuse not to work out, doesn't that same phrase come to mind?

Leading an active lifestyle—both in the bedroom and beyond—is very much a part of life, or *should* be, at least. Those who report being the happiest and healthiest of people typically enjoy their sex lives and participate in a variety of physical activities that keep them fit. It's not that sex and exercise go hand in hand all the time (or that you get enough of both), but these two components to life have direct connections to our moods, general psychology, and sense of vitality. They also share close ties to sleep.

Sex Just Gets More Complicated

Talking about the quality of one's sex life used to be taboo—something you didn't dare discuss at cocktail parties or around the office water cooler. But then Viagra hit the market and became the hottest new drug in 1998. Suddenly, it was okay to talk candidly about sexual dysfunction and the quality (and quantity) of one's sexual experience. Even women—who were not necessarily the targeted market for a drug like Viagra—wondered when they'd get their version. Some women demanded

Viagra from their doctors and started taking it, too. Obviously, both sexes had long been waiting for a magical pill to enhance their sex lives. Once again, I wish someone had asked me about the best way to boost a sex life.

When something about sex gets "discovered" by a scientific method (or close enough), it's widely reported. I remember when an Italian research team headed by a sexologist found that couples who have a TV set in their bedroom have sex half as often as those who don't. The psychologists questioned 523 Italian couples to see what effect television had on their sex lives. While the size of the study group probably isn't large enough to make any overall definitive conclusion, it certainly gives one pause to think about the total impact having a television in the bedroom has—affecting both sleep *and* sex.

But if it's not the television that inhibits regular lovemaking, lack of sleep surely does. And we've got a survey to prove it: According to the National Sleep Foundation's 2005 poll, nearly a quarter of couples in the United States admit to being so sleepy that they have lost interest in lovemaking. Those who snore also appear to have inferior sex lives, as the survey pointed out that more than a third of respondents say snoring causes a problem in the relationship. How many times have you slept in a separate bed, bedroom, or on the couch to avoid a bad bed partner? How much does that setup affect your level of intimacy? Probably more than you'd like to realize if you're among those who keep separate nighttime quarters for the sake of a good night's sleep.

If you've tried all of the methods I suggest in the Action Plan for couples, and you've done your best to customize your bedroom setting to you and your partner's specifications, then sleeping in separate rooms might be an option. But it should be the solution of last resort. There's something to be said for the intimate bond that gets reinforced when a couple sleeps together. And if you begin to go your separate ways at nighttime, you never know where that might lead you from a psychological standpoint. The physical separation might slowly erode your emotional connection, thus causing bigger problems down the road than you ever anticipated. I have often said that I've saved more marriages as a sleep specialist than I would have as a marital therapist, simply by getting people back in the bedroom together again.

About a quarter of partnered adults frequently sleep solo because they don't sleep well with their loved one. The most common problems are a partner's snoring and restlessness. This percentage doesn't even include those who choose to sleep alone due to mismatched schedules or preferences like temperature and mattress firmness. A National Sleep Foundation survey found that troubling bedmates steal forty-nine minutes of sleep away from their partners, on average, each night. For some couples, keeping separate quarters works, but for others, it cuts deeply into a relationship's intimacy.

Joe never thought he'd be the victim of a sexless life due to poor sleep. He came to me because his wife said he snored and it was keeping her awake a night, but that wasn't what he was worried about most. Joe found that he was so tired each evening that once the lights were out, so was he. When he thought about sex he had to negotiate with himself, and usually wound up thinking, Okay, tomorrow night. If I just get some rest tonight, I'll have more energy and be able to at least be more interested tomorrow.

These thoughts went on for months. Joe and his wife had had a healthy sex life once upon a time, but it had declined significantly over the years. Now Joe felt resentful that he and his wife were not having sex more often. In the rare moments when he wasn't tired, his wife was.

I brought them both into the clinic and when we talked we discovered several different things. First, Joe had some signs of sleep apnea: He was snoring, he was tired, and his wife had heard him gasp for breath a few times at night. That one was a no-brainer; I ordered him to participate in a sleep study to determine if he had sleep apnea, which he did. Questioning his wife, Colleen, also revealed that she had sleep problems as well. She was worried about Joe. She had seen one of my articles on WebMD.com and thought her husband might have some issues. And his snoring was so loud that it intruded on the quality of her own sleep, sapping her desire to be intimate.

Joe and Colleen experienced an amazing transformation. Once we identified Joe's apnea and worked hard on a treatment solution for him, Colleen's stress decreased and she no longer had to listen to his snoring. Within a month they were both reporting feeling much more alive and alert during the day. They were getting a good night's sleep routinely and the opportunities to engage in sex were happening much more frequently now because neither one would complain of being too tired. I was very pleased by how much marital strife they'd successfully sent away.

The timing of sex between two people who don't share the same sleep schedule can be another big hurdle to clear. But before we get to that, let's take a closer look at how sleep and sex work together.

HOW DOES SLEEP AFFECT SEX DRIVE?

Think about it: What causes you to want to have sex? Usually, there are some external stimuli or internal thoughts that cause a cascade of hormones (estrogen and testosterone) to increase blood pressure and heart rate, tighten muscles, and cause brain chemicals (neurotransmitters) to go into overdrive. But with women it's not that simple (which is partly why there is no magic "blue pill" for women). A couple's drive to have sex is incredibly complicated, involving biology as well as factors including the quality of the relationship, age, emotional health, medications, and attitudes about sex. Any one or combination of these factors can affect sex drive. Complicating matters is the fact that arousal is different from drive. Arousal is the physical ability to get your body to actually have sex. So you can have the drive but the incapacity to get aroused easily. And this can be a hindrance to experiencing satisfactory sex.

Sex should be an enjoyable experience with a partner, but here's a common experience:

> I was just so tired all the time. Between carpools, the baby, and life on the run, I was just too tired for sex. And when we did have sex, it wasn't like it used to be. I felt like I was going through the motions but, I hate to say it, not really there. My husband was getting frustrated, and I think it was affecting our marriage. I felt that if I could just get some good sleep, many other things would fall into place.

A low sex drive is the most common sexual complaint made by women—up to 30 percent to 40 percent of women. Although there is little research in this area, here are five facts we know about sleep that can translate to issues with sex. You be the judge:

First, lack of sleep causes increased moodiness, depression, and anxiety. These are all emotions that affect your drive for sex. Second, lack of sleep slows basic thinking processes. If you are not thinking straight, you may say or do something that can damage the moment. Third, lack of sleep slows reaction time. Being lethargic in bed is never a turn-on. Fourth, increased stress usually means less time for both sleep and sex. Finally, lack of sleep from several sleep disorders has been demonstrated to cause certain levels of sexual dysfunction. And, to top it off, as previously noted, many snoring bed partners find themselves sleeping alone.

In a British survey conducted by the British Snoring & Sleep Apnea Association, more than 60 percent of participants said they would make love more often if they or their partner stopped snoring. Most of the suffering partners were not the men—they were the women.

Sara W.'s story presents a classic case of how making a few adjustments in the bedroom can revive a sex life. Sara was a working mom with a lot on her shoulders. She and her husband were under constant financial stress, and when the pressures got really bad, Sara's old battle with insomnia resurfaced. What made it worse was her husband's snoring, which became chronic and very disruptive to Sara's sleep. As he gained weight, the snoring worsened to the point that Sara sometimes slept out on the couch. If she didn't fall asleep before he did (when he'd start snoring), she knew she'd never get to sleep and those anxious feelings would fuel the insomnia. Her solution was to either get into bed very early, pop in some earplugs, and hope for the best, or wait until the first phase of his snoring ceased and then climb into bed. Needless to say, they didn't have much time to be intimate while planning their sleep schedules around his snoring.

Sara wasn't a hopeless case. As it turned out, her husband suffered from terrible allergies that resulted in constant nasal congestion. After a trip to his doctor and some prescription nasal sprays, his congestion got quite a bit better and he slept better. In addition, we changed his tired old pillow (which was full of allergens and dust mites), and voilà . . . he had better sleep. Then he lost some weight, and the snoring went away. Sara immediately began sleeping better and her insomnia vanished. With both of them getting sound sleep, they experienced more energy and no longer had to schedule their bedtimes differently. This, in turn, automatically enhanced the frequency—and quality—of their sex.

HOW DOES SEX AFFECT SLEEP?

Sex definitely affects men and women differently, especially after orgasm. An anonymous person shares an experience that is common among women:

> After he has an orgasm, he is out cold. I don't know if it's the physical act of him having sex and orgasm, the afterglow, or what, but he's in la-la land and I'm ready to clean the house! It's so frustrating to sit there and watch him sleep. I would often turn on the TV and he would wake up, saying, "What are you doing still up?" with a dazed look on his face.

To understand this different postcoital experience, here are the theories. When a woman approaches orgasm, several chemicals in the brain begin to rise. Some of these chemicals (specifically, oxytocin, which is often called the "cuddle" hormone, and norepinephrine, the "alertness" hormone) are received by the brain at full speed. This may make a woman seek social contact or want to become more active.

The period of time for a woman to reach an orgasm is longer than in her male partner, so while she may be just getting started, her partner may already be on the downward slope. In addition, her levels of arousal will stay high for longer periods of time (hence the ability to have multiple orgasms), but this may also interfere with the ability to sleep.

Another factor may be the type of sex you are having: sensual versus vigorous or aerobic. It should come as no surprise that sex and exercise are quite similar activities. As we will discuss in the next section, increased aerobic effort can cause endorphins to kick in and, over time (four to six hours), they can cause a calming effect. This is why we think daytime exercise helps nighttime sleep. But when was the last time you saw an Olympic athlete take a nap after the 100-meter dash? Not likely. Increased aerobic sex just before bed is often arousing, while romantic and sensual sex may tend to be more relaxing. I am not suggesting that you avoid aerobic sex, but you can consider when you do it so that it will not not affect your sleep if you notice this is a problem.

Sexual tension, or the urge to have sex, may also make it difficult to fall asleep. Trying to go to bed and fall asleep while sexually aroused is an impossible task for many. (This is when self-stimulation can help, but again, it needs to be more relaxed and controlled than an aerobic event.) Men have such high levels of testosterone in their brain that it can buffer— neutralize—the effects of the cuddle hormone. This might explain why some women like to cuddle after sex, whereas some men do not.

Where's the research? Unfortunately, few studies review the effects of sex on sleep. Although one study showed no difference in post-climax sleepiness between men and women, I say the anecdotal evidence is far too strong to ignore. Ask most women and you'll find they stay aroused after sex. My clinical experience where I spend time with patients, and listen to hundreds of women's personal stories, attests to this fact. When I address the topic of sex with my female patients, most of them share that once their partner has had an orgasm, he is usually done for the night. Many of those men will then fall sleep almost minutes after reaching orgasm. The women, however, have an opposite response. They report feeling energized after they've reached orgasm, especially if they've had more than one. Although the technical research does not support these ideas, I think it's safe to say that this may be occurring in more bedrooms than not.

Other reasons that explain why men fall asleep after sex include: They were tired to begin with; the muscle tension released after orgasm has a relaxing effect; the increases in core body temperature and the subsequent drop in body temperature may trigger the brain chemical melatonin; or the decreases in oxygen during the act itself makes them sleepy. But we really don't know.

How can sex make you look younger? A large-scale, ten-year study performed by Dr. David Weeks in the 1990s at the Royal Edinburgh Hospital in Scotland found that sex helps you look between four and seven years younger. Dr. Weeks interviewed more than 3,500 people aged 18 to 102 in Britain, Europe, and the U.S. Dr. Weeks attributes this finding to significant reductions in stress, greater contentment, and better sleep. No surprise there.

Both men and women have a sexual response to sleep, specifically during REM (rapid eye movement) stages of sleep. In fact, your brain is as active during REM sleep as it is when you're awake. Both genders show engorgement of the erectile tissue during REM, and this is when you're likely to have sexual dreams. Since we know from research that REM sleep increases toward the end of the evening, this may explain those early morning feelings of desire. Testosterone levels are greatest in the A.M., which can lead to those amorous feelings as well.

HOW DOES BETTER SLEEP PROMOTE BETTER SEX?

As you've already learned from Chapter 5, your body secretes certain hormones during sleep, many of which can affect sex drive. For example, during the night, your body pumps out DHEA (dehydroepiandrosterone), which helps produce the sexual hormones testosterone and estrogen. Without these two hormones, you wouldn't have much of a drive at all.

The other two big factors are energy and emotions. Sleep is what allows us to boost our energy and moods—two essential ingredients in a quality sex life. Plus, with proper rest we experience a decrease in the emotions that can decrease sexual drive, such as depression, anxiety, and irritability. And mood might be an underestimated element.

We all know how our sleep or lack of sleep can affect our mood. For example, how likely are you to get upset when you have had a good night's sleep versus when you have not? We can get grumpy, short-tempered, and in some cases, downright mean (and not like our normal selves). The scary thing is sometimes we won't even realize it. Now think about this: How often do you get "in the mood" when you are sleep deprived? Is it more or less than normal? Another interesting notion: If you have said something to your partner because you are sleep deprived and in a bad mood, even if you do want to become intimate, how likely do you think he or she is going to be to return those feelings?

Another way to look at this situation is to consider what good sleep can do for your mood. Substantial research shows that in people with acute, chronic, and partial sleep deprivation, if they get better rest, their mood becomes markedly elevated. I hypothesize that this translates to better sexual activity. These results aren't all that astounding: If you're in a good mood, you'll likely be able to get "in the mood."

Tips to Matching Two Different Schedules for Sex

She's the owl and he's the lark. She goes to bed two to three hours after he does, and he gets up about two to three hours before she does. She prefers sex at night, whereas he likes it in the morning. How can these two different people ever come together for sex at the same time? After all, a deficit in physical affection can cause more tension than just the other responsibilities (and stresses) of home life, such as kids and balancing work and play.

Finding that intersection that happily meets the needs of both partners and doesn't result in anyone making a huge sacrifice (of sleep!) can be tough. This is when you might have to get crafty with scheduling sex. Here are some ideas:

- Be open and honest about your needs. Communicate.
- Make reservations. Pick a night, or two. Decide together which nights are best, considering both your schedules and your children's. Be realistic but make a commitment. Be open to *some* compromise.
- Defend the times you pick and treat them as sacred moments that will strengthen your partnership.
- Do what you need to do to avoid fatigue on your scheduled night. For example, pamper yourself that evening and avoid the task of preparing a large dinner and cleaning the kitchen. Anticipate the activity and mentally prepare. If you usually work until after 7:00, aim to leave the office earlier and don't say yes to a working dinner with colleagues or associates.
- If financially feasible, consider leaving the kids to babysitters more often, to enjoy a date night with your spouse once a week and a full getaway weekend once a month.
- Schedule sex during atypical times that work well no matter who's the lark or who's the owl, such as weekend afternoons.
- Savor the times you *can* be spontaneous with your partner. Those moments do arise on occasion. Grab them when you can!

Exercise and Sleep

I'm not the first person to tell you that exercise is good for you. But if there's one magic bullet for enhancing the quality of your life—from increasing your overall health to fighting the onset of age-related disease and elevating your mood and sense of well-being—it's exercise. And it can also have a positive impact on your sleep.

A book about the benefits of exercise is, well, a book in itself. You should be engaging in a physical activity at least thirty minutes or more five days a week (preferably six) that gets your heart rate up and makes you breathe a little harder. You don't have to go out and start training for a marathon, but you do need to work out at an intensity that challenges your cardiorespiratory fitness level and increases circulation. In addition to your cardiovascular workouts you should also think about strength training, which typically involves weight-bearing exercises, to build muscle mass, promote bone formation, and prevent bone loss. Stretching exercises that improve your flexibility are also important.

For the beginner, starting an exercise routine is hard. The good news is you can get a lot out of just going for a brisk thirty-minute walk every day and buying a couple of free weights to use after you get back and perform some post-walking stretches. Several studies have suggested that walking can be just as good as jogging.

Exercise can add three years to life expectancy. Those extra years are attributed largely to the avoidance of heart disease, which is the number one killer in America for both men and women.

Because sleep and exercise are both vital signs of good health, if you can accomplish both well, you're way ahead of the game.

If you can engage in regular physical activity most days of the week, you automatically reduce the risk of developing or dying from some of the leading causes of illness and death in the United States. Exercise:

- lowers the risk of heart disease.
- lowers the risk of diabetes.
- lowers the risk of high blood pressure.
- lowers the risk of colon cancer.
- lowers feelings of depression and anxiety.
- lowers risk of stroke, dementia, and Alzheimer's disease.
- lowers back pain and risk of osteoporosis.
- helps control weight.

- helps manage stress.
- helps build and maintain healthy bones, muscles, and joints.
- promotes psychological well-being.
- *makes you look and feel younger!*

Now, imagine a pill you could take that does all that. Exercise is exactly that pill.

Bonus: If you suffer from high blood pressure, high cholesterol, diabetes, arthritis, or depression, exercise can reduce the severity of your condition.

THE SLEEP BENEFITS TO AEROBIC EXERCISE

To reap the sleep benefits of exercise, stretching and lifting weights won't do the trick. Even though those exercises are good for you, they should supplement exercise that strengthens your cardiovascular system, such as running, swimming, bicycling, skiing, playing tennis, and even walking to a step aerobics class at the gym.

Not everyone experiences the same sleep benefits to exercise, but people who suffer from insomnia aren't usually the athletes and highly active individuals. (The only instance I've seen is where athletes overtrain and for some reason have a hard time turning their mind off at night, or they are so used to exercising that on their "off days" their body craves that exercise to help with sleep.) To the contrary, most people who complain of sleep problems lead sedentary lives and don't practice a regular exercise routine. Aerobic exercise has been shown to aid in sleep primarily by doing two things: 1) helping you fall asleep quicker; and 2) plunging you into deep (or delta) sleep for a longer period of time, which is where you need to be to feel refreshed and restored the next day. Studies on people who participate in aerobic activities show that they have a tendency to secrete more growth hormone at night, which aids in repairing and rejuvenating the body.

One of the current ideas behind exercise's effects on sleep centers of the brain is the thermogenic hypothesis, which states that exercise promotes sleep by heating the body or brain. When you work out (again, it has to be an aerobic workout for at least twenty to thirty minutes), your body's core temperature rises a couple of degrees (about 2 degrees

Fahrenheit) and stays that way for about four to five hours. When it cools back down, your core temperature will decrease to a point lower than had you not worked out at all. And it's this drop in body temperature that is theorized to promote going to sleep more quickly as well as deep, sound sleep.

Throughout this book you'll learn details about sleep-wake rhythms as dictated by light, temperature, and activity. Briefly, your circadian rhythm is defined by cycles of temperature and exposure to light every day. If you're a day worker who sleeps at night and is awake during the daylight hours, your body temperature goes up during the day and down at night, bottoming out sometime in the very early morning hours. It also takes a slight dip in the early afternoon, which brings on that after-lunch lull. Exposure to bright light, especially that from sunlight, plays a critical role in naturally resetting your rhythm every day so your sleep-wake cycles remain stable. Physical activity can act like light in this regard, helping set and maintain your biological clock naturally. The question is, however, when should you schedule that physical activity so you get those sleep benefits at the right time?

The answer to that question, unfortunately, is that it *depends*. Some argue that because of the four-to-five-hour temperature boost after exercise and subsequent fall, the best time is about five to six hours before bedtime. And that you can't exercise strenuously just prior to bed while your temperature is still up. The benefits to exercise are so strong that I don't think it should really matter what time of day you find time to exercise, so long as you do it. In other words, it's hard enough to worry about fitting the time in to schedule a workout than it is to time it perfectly. During the 28-night program you'll have the opportunity to experiment with working out at different times of the day. If exercise arouses you for a very long time, thus intruding upon your sleep, then you'll have to schedule your workouts earlier in the day. If, however, exercise has nothing but sleep-promoting effects on you, then feel free to work out later in the day. After-work hours are often very popular times.

The effects temperature has on our bodies for sleep purposes also explain how a hot tub, sauna, or warm bath can aid us in falling asleep easily and achieving more slow-wave, deep sleep.

The average adult receives only about twenty minutes of daily exposure to bright light, which is defined as more than 2,500 lux. People who exercise regularly outdoors possibly receive at least three times this much exposure, thus augmenting the natural calibration of their circadian rhythms.

Keep in mind that the idea of exercise promoting sleep is variable to some extent. A lot depends on your individual body's physiology and even psychology. There's a lot to be said for exercise's ability to lower depression and encourage the release of mood-elevating endorphins. That "runner's high" you hear about is attributed to the surge of endorphins that accompanies a strenuous physical workout. What's more, the mood boost that exercise offers isn't limited to just during and right after your workout. Exercise is proven to enhance your overall sense of well-being, lowering your stress load and taking the wind out of those bedtime anxiety attacks that keep you up. Anxiety is, after all, perhaps the number one reason people can't get to sleep at night. By exercising at some point during the day, you might give yourself the "off" switch your mind needs to quickly drift toward dreamland.

How to Get the Most Out of Exercise's Benefits

- Get a physical and discuss your goals to get fit with your doctor, ruling out any medical issues you need to address in pursuit of establishing an exercise program.
- Experiment with exercise at different times of the day: First find a convenient time, and then worry about whether it disrupts your sleep or not.
- Include cardio training, strength training, and stretching for flexibility.
- Be sure to get your heart rate up for at least twenty to thirty minutes most days of the week.
- Build your fitness level slowly; don't jump into a strenuous fitness routine too quickly.
- Exercise in bright outdoor light if possible.

How much exercise will affect your sleep will be a result of the level of intensity at which you work out, how long you work out, as well as how fit you are to begin with. If you train too hard and stress your body maximally, those benefits can turn against you and exercise suddenly can become a sleep thief. Overtraining is seen a lot among serious athletes and fitness enthusiasts. Classic symptoms include persistent muscle soreness, fatigue, low energy, depression, and sleep disturbance.

How Sleep Affects Physical Performance

If I told you to pull an all-nighter the day before you're going to run the New York City Marathon, what do you think that sleepless night would do to your performance and ability to finish the race?

I know what you'd say—*my performance would plummet, and I'd have a really hard time finishing*—but the science to prove that isn't what you'd expect. And it's fuzzy.

Most athletes or non-athletes who like to recreationally compete think the interruption or loss of sleep may be the cause of decreased performance. Coaches and trainers preach the benefits of sleep, but here's a surprise: Lack of sleep doesn't appear to hurt physical endurance or strength. What science tells us is that sleep deprivation, such as staying up for thirty to sixty hours, has little or no effect on aerobic performance and respiratory factors.

However, there are a few exceptions to this rule. For example, exercise above 75 percent of your maximum effort should be preceded by a normal night's sleep in order to perform well. Why? The mental effects of sleep deprivation can have consequences. So even though you can physically run the same distance or lift the same weight on little sleep, the moodiness, anxiety, and irritability that accompanies your sleep debt will likely turn that run or weight-lifting session into a struggle.

People seem to think they are working harder during physical exercise (called perceived exertion) after sleep deprivation, but that's not necessarily true. Perceived exertion increases with sleep deprivation, but the key word here is *perceived*. People who have undergone sixty hours of sleep deprivation can react as fast, and with as much force, as those who have had seven hours of sleep per night.

To give sleep some credit here, exercisers do seem to get to a quitting point more quickly (called a reduced time to the point of exhaustion) while sleep deprived, and research has also found that there is a significant reduction in glucose tolerance after sleep deprivation, which can affect sustained aerobic exercise. There's some evidence that lack of sleep interferes with the metabolism of glucose, which the body depends on for recovery. But still, I am surprised that studies don't blatantly show that sleep deprivation cuts sharply into athletic performance. (Very little research has been done on the effect of sleep deprivation on anaerobic power and strength, such as weight lifting. Any results in this area of research also point to sleep deprivation having no effect.)

By now, you're thinking, Gee, so being sleep deprived has no effect on my capacity to perform physically! Not so fast. Many of the sleep-deprivation studies are done on people forced to stay up for at least thirty hours. When was the last time you stayed up for thirty-plus hours in a row? It's not a likely situation (hopefully), which is why I dug a bit deeper into the research on *partial* sleep deprivation. Partial sleep deprivation is what happens when you sleep poorly and get interrupted throughout the night by disturbances like a snoring partner or the need to use the bathroom.

The results of studies performed on people whose sleep patterns were interrupted, as opposed to being totally deprived of sleep, were completely different. To start, while partial sleep loss causes no reduction in maximal performance, it causes several physiological changes. Your hand steadiness declines, and so does your anaerobic power to lift weights. These declines do return to normal after a good night's sleep.

Olympic athletes don't scrimp on sleep. They know that it's not just about their physical performance; mental ability and emotional well-being can be bigger factors when it comes to winning at the Games. According to former NASA scientist Dr. Mark Rosekind, who helped prepare Team USA at the Olympic Training Facility in Colorado Springs prior to the Winter Games in Turin, Italy, in 2006, the proper amount of sleep can boost an athlete's performance as much as 30 percent. When it comes to performance, he also believes that two hours less sleep than needed is the same as having a blood-alcohol level of .05. You can bet he prioritized sleep high on the list of things to do in preparing those American athletes.

Finally, it's worth reminding you that lack of sleep can compromise the immune system, which can be vulnerable already during hard physical training and bouts of intense exercise. Though science can't explain all the mechanisms in complete detail, research shows that sleep deprivation alters the activity of the body's killer cells. For example, sleep loss around the time of vaccination for influenza has been shown to reduce the production of flu-fighting antibodies. Keeping your sleep bank filled may also help fight cancer, a fairly recent finding that I'll detail in Chapter 11. So getting adequate sleep will bolster your immune system and further support your active lifestyle.

WHAT DOES THIS ALL MEAN?

The research to support theories that sleep deprivation negatively affects exercise may not be very convincing, but that's not what should concern you. Sleep deprivation has a great psychological effect on the mind because your perceived exertion after a bad night's sleep is enough to diminish the quality of your exercise—if you find the energy to exercise at all. In other words, you expect your workout to be more difficult, and, as such, it is. Any decline in performance after sleep deprivation is more than likely brought about by psychological expectations.

Feeling tired and cranky is enough to get you to say, "I'm too tired to exercise," so the real question is: How can you increase your energy for exercise and get the most out of your workout? Sleep.

Although it was originally thought that exercise before bed could negatively impact sleep, some research shows that in anxious individuals, exercise before bed can be quite calming. You'll learn how to experiment with timing exercise right during the 28-night program.

CHAPTER 7

Time-Out: Naps, Siestas, and Kips

Naps are good for you.

Naps are bad for you.

Naps will alleviate daytime sleepiness, recharge your energy, and not affect your nighttime slumber.

Naps will make you groggy and drowsy the rest of the day and will rob you of a good night's sleep.

What's the truth about naps?

They call them siestas in Spain and kips in England. Whatever you call the mid-day snooze, napping has been controversial from a scientific standpoint for quite some time. Some books (and their authors) will tell you to avoid naps entirely during the day or risk another sleepless night. Others contend naps—when timed properly—will enhance your alertness in the afternoon, increase your ability to concentrate, and assist you in achieving sound sleep at night.

There is no iron-clad answer to the napping question except to say people respond as differently to naps as they do to the number of hours slept. I do, however, think that more people could benefit from experimenting with naps and making time for them. In this chapter, we're going to take a look at the art of napping and what you can do to see whether or not you're the type who can reap enormous rewards from getting a little shut-eye during the day. There are, of course, rules or guidelines to napping, which I'll cover.

Naps have been gaining popularity (and acceptance in the work-place) ever so slowly. In fact, in 2004, the first MetroNaps facility opened in New York City's Empire State Building, which offers uniquely designed "Pods" for sneaking in a power nap during the day. (Funny how the term *power nap* has replaced *cat nap*, as if that's a more accept-able phrase.) The Pods, which look like something out of a James Bond movie, block sound and light and offer the perfect micro-environment for various lengths of naps. Similar to gyms and spas, these MetroNaps facilities offer passes you can use for frequent visits. Another such MetroNaps facility can be found in Vancouver's International Airport, where travelers can catch a snooze before or in between flights. It will be interesting to see just how far this idea can go, and if someday we'll see such sleeping Pods filling a room at a company's headquarters or lo-cated in a store on a corner next to a Starbucks. Imagine a day when taking a nap is as trendy as taking a coffee break or going out to lunch. Some companies do have designated napping areas that aren't quite as fancy as a place like MetroNaps, but they do offer rooms with comfort-able recliners, soft lighting, music, and an overall soothing atmosphere.

Millions of adults are supplementing their sleep with naps. More than half of adult Americans nap at least once a week, and one-third nap twice a week. The average nap lasts fifty minutes. The National Sleep Foundation reports that 33 percent of adults surveyed would nap at work, if allowed.

Winston Churchill said: "You must sleep sometime between lunch and dinner, and no halfway measures. Take off your clothes and get into bed. That's what I always do."

The Pros of Napping

Forget what you might have heard in the past about naps. For those who respond well to naps (and who learn the ropes to perfecting this art), naps can provide a wealth of rewards that go beyond just making you feel better and able to tackle the rest of your day. Naps have been shown scientifically to benefit almost every aspect of human wellness—from the physical rewards of lowering your risk for heart disease and repairing cells to the more obvious ones of lifting your mood and stamina, knocking down stress, and making you more productive. Because naps can improve heart functioning, support hormonal maintenance, and encourage cell repair, they can help you live longer, stay more active, and look younger. These benefits, of course, are what nocturnal sleep is for, so the purpose of a nap is to plunge you into and out of rejuvenating sleep as fast as possible. By doing so, you tap into these benefits during the day instead of having to wait until nighttime to recoup them. The ultimate result? MRIs of nappers have shown that brain activity stays high throughout the day with a nap; without one, it declines as the day wears on.

> Famous nappers include Albert Einstein, Thomas Edison, Leonardo da Vinci, Napoleon Bonaparte, Ronald Reagan, Bill Clinton, and many others. Brahms napped at the piano while composing his famous lullaby. Winston Churchill scheduled his cabinet meetings around his naps, alleging that he required a daily afternoon nap in order to cope with his wartime responsibilities. Some of today's top athletes and Olympians take long naps in the afternoons as part of their training regimen. Their naps are as important as their daily exercise. Cyclist Lance Armstrong's coach, Chris Carmichael, admits, "Naps were critical in his overall training plan."

The brain is the part of the body most affected by a nap, which is evidenced by a greater alertness, improved memory retention, and enhanced ability to think creatively and insightfully. By sharpening your motor skills and neuromuscular coordination, napping can make you better at just about anything you do, from dancing and playing the piano to driving a car, making quick decisions, responding to stimuli or danger, exploring the Internet, and typing frantically on a computer or a BlackBerry.

Psychologist Dr. Sara C. Mednick, a scientist at the Salk Institute for Biological Studies in San Diego, has been leading the way in conducting napping research, publishing convincing data with colleagues at Harvard University, among others, on the value and benefits of napping. Collectively, recent findings among the top nap researchers are demonstrating just how naps enhance information processing and learning. In a nutshell, napping has been shown to:

- improve a person's capacity to learn certain tasks, and
- reverse information overload by protecting brain circuits from overuse until those neurons can consolidate what's already been learned.

In one particular study, reported in the July 2002 issue of *Nature Neuroscience*, Mednick and her colleagues at Harvard University demonstrated that "burnout"—irritation, frustration, and poorer performance on a mental task—sets in as a day wears on. In the study, subjects performed a visual task that tested their ability to concentrate and respond quickly. Their scores on the task worsened over the course of four daily practice sessions. Allowing subjects a thirty-minute nap after the second session prevented any further deterioration, while a one-hour nap actually boosted performance in the third and fourth sessions back to morning levels. This study also showed that a 20 percent overnight improvement in learning a motor skill is largely traceable to a late stage of sleep that you might be missing if you're an early riser. What's more, the research suggests that the brain uses a night's sleep to consolidate the memories of habits, actions, and skills learned during the day.

So, in essence, nighttime sleep and mid-day naps can go hand in hand. And if you can nap long enough to cycle through slow-wave (or deep) sleep, you can awaken ahead of everyone else who's burned out from their day. In fact, the recent research is raising the profile of slow-wave sleep as a possible means by which naps might foster learning.

> For people with narcolepsy, naps are especially important. A nap can actually replace a dosage of a stimulant medication.

THE REASONING BEHIND THAT AFTERNOON LULL

It's 2 P.M. You've just had lunch and you're trying to get back to work for a productive afternoon. But you feel as if someone is swinging a hypnotic pendulum in front of your eyes. You're drowsy, barely able to stay awake and keep your mind focused on anything but sleep. In fact, you're already daydreaming about resting your head down on the desk and shutting your eyes for a brief moment. What's happening?

A lot is happening, actually. In the next chapter you're going to learn how to define the profile of your natural sleep pattern by timing when you hit that afternoon lull. It's all a part of your body's biological, circadian rhythm that defines your sleep-wake cycles, which you'll recall I mentioned briefly before. Similar to your body's drop in temperature and level of alertness at night, you also experience a smaller drop in core body temperature and alertness in the middle of the day, typically twelve hours after the middle of your night's rest or roughly eight hours after awakening.

Don't be too quick to blame your afternoon coma on your heavy lunch (or, as some say, "food coma"). If you feel sluggish and sleepy just after lunch, it's most likely because your body is naturally cycling through its twenty-four-hour sleep rhythm, which causes it to mimic slightly how it is in the middle of the night—regardless of what you ate or drank at lunch. A human's natural sleep pattern is biphasic, so twice during a twenty-four-hour period we all experience a drop in core body temperature that invites sleep. From a cultural perspective, this is probably why siestas came to be.

It's really true: Research has shown that taking a twenty-minute nap about eight hours after your wake time can do more for you than hitting that snooze button for another twenty minutes in the morning. The recuperative effects of a nap that lasts less than thirty minutes have been confirmed. What's more, it's also been confirmed that a short nap containing three minutes of Stage II sleep has recuperative effects, whereas these effects are limited following only Stage I sleep.

HOW LONG IS THE PERFECT NAP?

The twenty-minute power nap has been talked about for years, but napping doesn't have to be so confined. You can gain a lot of benefits from as little as five minutes, and as much as two or more hours (but, please, no more than three). As mentioned earlier, if you can achieve a full cycle of sleep through slow-wave, or deep, sleep, you stand to gain the most out of a mid-day snooze.

When billionaire adventurer Steve Fossett broke the record for the around-the-world solo jet flight in the spring of 2005, he slept just sixty minutes in sixty-seven hours of flight time. Those sixty minutes were broken into two- and three-minute naps. He reported that none of his feats could have been accomplished without these micro-variety power naps.

If you've tried to nap in the past and you've awakened groggy and feeling worse off than beforehand, this is most likely because you haven't timed it right and you've awakened in the middle of that slow-wave sleep stage. During this stage, your brain's activity is polar opposite to how it functions while you're awake. At this stage, you've completely tuned out the external world and your entire brain rhythm synchronizes into a slow, uniform pattern instead of multitasking and operating on many frequencies. If you suddenly come out of slow-wave sleep, you force your brain to desynchronize and fire off high-frequency electrical activity. Until your brain catches up to the fact you're actually awake, you'll feel slow, sleepy, and probably cranky, too. Your limbs will feel like heavyweights, your eyes won't focus well, you'll have a hard time sounding articulate, and your mind will feel left behind. A quick way to slap your brain into wakeful shape is to do something physical, listen to stimulating music, or splash cold water on your face.

Sleep inertia is that undeniable feeling of grogginess upon awakening that temporarily reduces your ability to perform even simple tasks. It can last from one minute to four hours, but typically lasts only fifteen to thirty minutes . . . and can be reversed with activity, noise, and light. The severity of sleep inertia depends on how long you've been asleep and which stage of sleep you were in upon awakening.

The Architecture of Sleep

Understanding the value of a nap comes with understanding your sleep cycles. As you're probably already aware, when you go to bed at night, your brain doesn't become flatlined and you're not resting in the same "state" all night long. There is a defined "architecture" to sleep that entails five distinct stages during which your brain's activity changes. These stages recur cyclically throughout your sleep. Stage I, the initial stage you enter soon after you start drifting and sinking toward feeling asleep, is when your brain's electrical activity slows, as does respiration, eye and jaw-muscle movement. Stage II features a light but restful sleep in which your body prepares for deep sleep by lowering temperature and relaxing muscles further. Stages III and IV are when you enter that deep slow-wave sleep. Stage V is the most famous stage of all—REM, when your eyes twitch and dreaming can become intense.

- Slow-wave (deep) sleep—Stages III and IV—is for restoring your *body*. This is when the release of growth hormone reaches a twenty-four-hour high.
- REM sleep—Stage V—is for restoring your *mind*. This is when specific neural connections are made, thus supporting the retention and organization of information as well as the shoring up of space to learn and perform new tasks.

These five sleep stages repeat every eighty to 120 minutes for a total of between four and six cycles a night. (The time from your first step downward into sleep to the end of the first REM sleep is called the first sleep cycle, and the time from then on to the end of the second REM sleep is the second sleep cycle.) Stage I can last from half a minute up to ten minutes, but doesn't provide many benefits from a restorative stand-point. Stage II, however, is the stage that nappers aim to reach because it's the gateway to Stage III and features a less intense form of delta sleep. (Stages III and IV are characterized by the brain emitting very low-frequency, high-voltage delta waves.) This is when your body has a chance to refresh itself. In addition to generally improving alertness and stamina, Stage II is marked by certain electrical signals in the nervous system that seem to solidify the connection between neurons involved in muscle memory. What this means is your neurons can act faster and with more accuracy after you've awakened.

THE GOAL OF NAPPING

The goal of a nap, then, is to dip the body and mind briefly into Stage II, which can last for twenty minutes (hence, the twenty-minute power nap) and then pull out quickly before lowering far into the deeper sleep of Stages III and IV. If you reach that slow-wave deep sleep, however, and don't wait until you cycle out of those lower stages, you'll experience sleep inertia. The solution to avoiding sleep inertia is to either time your nap carefully and keep it to twenty minutes or slightly less, or cycle all the way through and lengthen the nap to about fifty minutes.

The Cons of Napping

Although everyone is capable of napping, it's not going to be the magic bullet for conquering sleepiness during the day or fighting insomnia for everyone. This is why you have to be your own sleep therapist and experiment with a few types of naps (we'll go through these shortly). Napping is nearly impossible for a lot of people today, for many reasons, not the least of which include work commitments, no access to a suitable place to nap at the right time, and the typical stimulants running through the bloodstream during the day. For example, if the perfect time for you to nap is, say, 1:00 in the afternoon but you've just downed a grande latte and a Snickers bar (on top of three diet sodas in the morning), all that sugar and caffeine is going to work against you when you try to settle into a nap.

Napping will not interfere with your nighttime sleep so long as you get that nap in four to five hours before your bedtime. The nap should be less than three hours as well (this probably doesn't apply to you because, for most, having time for even a one-hour nap is a luxury).

Types of Naps

1. The twenty-minute **Power Nap.** Give yourself thirty minutes total, so you have ten minutes to prepare to fall asleep.
2. The sixty-to-ninety minute **Restorative Nap.** This nap takes you

through a full cycle of sleep, dipping you into slow-wave, deep sleep. Because reaching those lower stages (Stages III and IV) takes longer, you have to set aside ample time for your body to reach deep sleep and then come out. For most people, this equals about fifty minutes from the time you fall asleep. Achieving deep sleep is how your body truly restores itself, making this nap the most rejuvenating type of all.

3. **The Caf-Nap** (a.k.a. the Jump-start Your Engine Nap). As outlined in the Action Plan for the Caffeine fiend, drink a cup of drip coffee or caffeinated tea (medium warmth, not very hot, because you're going to guzzle it down) and then sleep in a reclining position. Be careful not to lie down flat on your back because acid reflux can occur. You'll wake up just in time for the caffeine to kick in and get the double whammy of alertness. (As previously mentioned, if you respond quickly to caffeine—shorter than the usual twenty minutes—this may not work for you.)

How do you know which nap to use and when? Take this quiz to find out.

QUIZ

1) **Are you a shift worker, or are you planning on working all night on a project?**

➤ If the answer is yes to either question, then you will require the preemptive Restorative Nap (sixty to ninety minutes) before you go into work or before you begin to work when the rest of the office has left (likely around 6:30 or 7 P.M.). You'll be asking your body to stay awake when it wants to sleep, and if you wait too long to take your nap, you'll run into the body's natural tendency to sleep for the entire night and it will be *extremely* difficult to wake up. A caveat: If you suffer from insomnia in any form, I would stay away from this type of nap.

2) **Are you napping because you didn't get enough sleep last night (fewer than five hours) and you need to be awake at work or school?**

➤ If the answer is yes, then you will want the twenty-minute Power Nap, which will have a nice restorative effect. Aim for scheduling the nap at about 11:30 to 12:00, giving yourself ten minutes to fall asleep. When you wake up, go to the restroom and wash your face—first with warm water and then again with water as cold as you can stand. You'll look less tired. Then go on to lunch for some nourishment.

You can also try the twenty-minute Caf-Nap here as well. Again, schedule the nap for 11:30 A.M.

3) Is it late in the day and you are experiencing the "afternoon lull"?

If yes, it may be best to avoid napping and, instead, go for a walk outside and get a little sunlight. Take the stairs to the outside and walk for a total of ten minutes. This should help quite a bit. If it doesn't, then the twenty-minute Power Nap is in order. Be careful about going for a Caf-Nap, which, depending on how late in the day it is, can encroach on your ability to fall asleep at bedtime.

The Rules to Napping

- Find a good napping place that's devoid of phones, loud noises, or disruptive people.
- Avoid direct sunlight while napping.
- Take off your shoes, and loosen your belt if it's tight.
- Try to nap in a reclined position either at your desk in a chair that swivels back so you can put your feet up, on the floor or couch, or in your car (but be safe).
- Be careful about the room temperature. You may need a blanket to stay warm since sleep drops your body temperature.
- Avoid napping past 3 P.M. It's better to nap according to your circadian rhythm, which for most means snoozing in the late morning or early afternoon. If you sleep later in the day, you face a higher risk of entering slow-wave deep sleep and emerging groggy.
- Watch what you eat and drink beforehand if you plan to nap. Anything high in fat, sugar, caffeine, or other stimulants can interrupt your nap time (unless you are going for the Caf-Nap). Go for calcium and protein within two hours of nap time.
- Use an alarm! Time your nap according to your needs.
- Once your nap is over, get up and walk outside, if possible. Absorbing sunlight will help with your circadian clock.
- Create a Napping Kit for optimal napping.

Your Napping Kit

1. eye shades
2. earplugs, or a digital music player with soft relaxing tunes
3. a light blanket
4. a travel-size neck pillow (U-shaped is best)
5. a small alarm clock or a wristwatch alarm

My Story

I love to nap. I don't allow it to replace my sleep, but I can supplement sleep after a particularly rough night up with the kids. In addition, I can also enjoy an early afternoon nap on the weekends when trying to get my children to nap as well.

When I first started my career I had just come out of graduate school and moved directly into my first "real job." I was working for a group of pulmonologists who had a four-bed sleep lab. I was told that my career with the group looked promising and I was expected to pass the medical board in sleep. I was a trained psychologist, though, not a medical doctor, so in order to take the exam I had to teach myself neurology, neurochemistry, pulmonology . . . and all the rest of the areas of medicine that would be on the test for sleep. I collected the requisite reading and set off on my merry way.

Every night, after a full day's work, I ventured to the Emory University Law Library for about three hours and read, made flash cards, and studied sleep medicine. I did this for about three straight months before the exam. At the same time, my fiancée and I were building a house and planning our wedding (which occurred three days after I took the boards). Needless to say, I was stressed, staying up late planning and studying. I certainly was not getting my requisite "sleep number" and was getting pretty tired during the day. Then I learned of the Caf-Nap idea and experimented with it. I saw patients in the mornings, and during lunch I closed my door, slugged a cup of coffee, and stole a twenty-minute nap. My nurse would then call me, wake me up, and I'd have lunch and be on my way. I can't tell you what a difference this made for me. Over time I got rid of the coffee and just did the Power Nap when I could and it always felt great. I also made sure that I had a backup alarm and a C-shaped pillow in my desk drawer. My naps always came in handy, despite quality sleep I was getting at home.

Next came the kids. When my wife had our first child, I thought I was prepared. Ha! Even though she was doing a majority of the work at night, I still woke up with almost every cry and when our little boy got sick, I would always try to be there. I've never been so sleep deprived in my entire life. At times my boss would look at me and say, "Mike, go back to the lab and lie down for a while, you need it," and he was right. As soon as I did this, I felt better and became more productive. I'll admit that naps haven't always been available to me. I can also say that when I have had the occasional time in my life where I was unable to sleep (due to insomnia-types of symptoms), napping was not a good option because it had direct effects on my ability to fall asleep during these hard times. But other than difficult or extra-stressful times in my life, I can happily say naps have been one of the most refreshing parts of my day.

Be patient with yourself as you learn how to nap and time your naps according to your body's needs. Napping is not a sign of being unmotivated and lazy. Quite the contrary, people who can nap successfully often lead more productive, healthier, and happier lives. They are less prone to errors at work, on the road, and in everyday activities.

SoundSleepSolutions.com

Don't forget to check out my Web site at www.soundsleepsolutions.com. There, you can write to me about your personal experiences with sleep, share your own tips on an active message board, and ask questions.

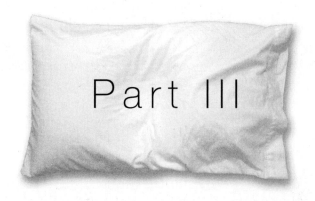

Part III

28 Nights to
Sound Sleep Forever

CHAPTER 8

Week 1: Your Sleep Boot Camp

I t's finally time to put your newly acquired sleep knowledge to a road test and see how twenty-eight nights can make a difference in your life. In the next month, you're going to perform little shifts in the way you approach sleep, and transform all the information you've learned up to this point (and probably tucked somewhere in your brain) into actual skills you practice regularly for life. If you successfully implemented the plans already outlined earlier in the book, congratulations. You're way ahead of the game; use this twenty-eight-night program to master those skills and build upon your sleep hygiene. If you kinda, sorta executed those Action Plans but feel the need for more structure in the form of a day-by-day program, you'll find exactly that starting in this chapter with step-by-step instructions, plus guidance for including those Action Plans.

Each day introduces a new focus or challenge, which you'll have to maintain throughout the twenty-eight nights. *This is a cumulative program that progresses each and every day.* What you do on the first day, for example, will still be addressed on the last day. Because most of the lifestyle modifications you'll be making have biological consequences, few of them can become routine overnight and, instead, will require work and vigilance over several weeks as your body adjusts and responds. This is what the twenty-eight nights are designed to allow. The best way to approach this chapter, as well as the subsequent chapters that guide you week by week, is to read through what's in the plans for an entire week. In other words, read Nights 1 through 7 at once, since the activities and goals will overlap. You may have to refer back to earlier parts in the book for more comprehensive instructions, but I'll tell you exactly when and where to go to do that.

If you follow this program diligently for twenty-eight nights, I guarantee that you'll "awaken" to a whole new you at the finish line. But let me be clear: This will be one of the hardest things you ever try to do. Why? Because you're going against ingrained habits that took years to create and could take a while to break. You've been conditioned to behave and act a certain way, and reconditioning those habits takes time, effort, and patience. Do not be discouraged if you don't complete the twenty-eight nights perfectly. (I'll suggest another option at the start of the next chapter if you cannot keep up and prefer to go a little slower, spreading out your program over the course of a longer period.) During this first week, however, try to keep with the given program; otherwise, the time it takes to see results lengthens.

For most, Week 1, which is outlined in this chapter, will seem the most intense as you're instructed to home in on your sleep habits and hygiene on several levels. But, hey, you have to start somewhere! The three weeks that follow are for reassessment, and personal tweaking so that the lifestyle modifications coincide to your individual needs.

Use the diary in Appendix A to record your progress and note the choices you make as you experiment with various aspects to sleep in this chapter and begin to formulate your own personal sleep habits. This diary is also available on my Web site in a free downloadable format at www.soundsleepsolutions.com. It will be essential that you record what I ask you to do, because in Week 2 we will be reviewing your progress based on these data. Remember to record everything and to be honest.

Week 1

NIGHT 1: ESTABLISH YOUR BEDTIME AND WAKE TIME

Figuring out the perfect bedtime and wake time for you will take more than just one day alone. This will be an ongoing experiment over the course of several days, maybe the entire month. By the eighth day (the beginning of Week 2), if you still feel like your sleep schedule isn't working, or you don't feel as well as you'd like to during the day, you'll have to experiment some more. This may entail creating some sleep deprivation so that sleep comes more easily, or playing with how many sleep cycles you schedule in each night. Take the experiments one day at a time. Keep in mind that we've got a full month to play with various scenarios, so be patient. Few sleep problems can be cured overnight.

> **Myth Buster:** *If you continue to not sleep well you will experience serious health problems.* Not true! This kind of thinking is called "catastrophic thinking," and it happens when you blow facts out of proportion. True, the research shows that if you sleep less than six hours a night consistently, you increase your *risk* for a variety of diseases such as colon cancer, breast cancer, heart disease, obesity, and diabetes (and probably getting run over by a bus because you can't pay attention). But you can't sleep deprive yourself to death. According to *Guinness World Records*, Randy Gardner set the record back in 1964, when the then-seventeen-year-old went eleven consecutive days (264 hours) without sleep. After staving off sleep for a few days with cold showers and loud music (not to mention media reporters and games of pinball), he could no longer focus his eyes and had to give up TV. His speech slurred, and he fell into a silent stupor. But he didn't die soon after. Guess what he did? He slept a little more than usual for a few nights. Sleep experts now believe that long, sleepless stints like Randy's can be dangerous, even though he paid back his sleep debt by getting extra sleep for a few nights, which earned him a normal, healthy, life again. The moral of the story: You can go for a period of time without quality sleep and experience the consequences. But you can recover quickly if you allow your body to recoup those lost hours again.

Before we determine exactly how many hours of sleep you need on average every night, and where sleep should be on your daily agenda, let's review a few facts:

1. The average adult sleeps less than seven hours a night during the workweek.

2. Twenty-six percent of men get fewer than six hours, while 17 percent of women get fewer than six hours.

3. The average person has five to six sleep cycles. Cycles average between 80 and 120 minutes. The first cycle lasts 70 to 100 minutes. The next four cycles are about 90 to 120 minutes each.

4. How sleepy you feel depends upon several factors: age, time of sleep, thoughts about sleep, diet, environmental factors (e.g., light, noise, exercise), and internal circadian rhythm.

One of the most essential pieces of information you need to achieve the best sleep habits is the number of times and for how long your sleep cycles last each night. Recall from Chapter 7 the basics about sleep cycles: Every night sleep comes via distinct stages that cycle through between four and six times during the night. These stages are based on the speed and amplitude of your brain waves. A "normal" sleep cycle occurs when you go from Stage I to Stages II, III, IV, back to II, and then into REM, which is where memory is consolidated, your body cannot move, and you're likely to dream. During REM, your brain's activity is similar to that of wakefulness. But you are clearly not awake. After REM, you descend again down through Stages II, III, and IV, and then ascend back up to REM. This descending and ascending from start to finish—beginning at Stage I and ending at REM—is called the sleep cycle.

Part of the goal of the following experiments is to figure out the profile of your sleep cycles. This is going to be a rough calculation, so don't approach this with expectations of total precision. Just do your best to arrive at the most realistic portrait of your night's sleep.

Many find that if they get a full five cycles during a night, they feel at their best the next day, so we'll use five as our target number.

Experiment #1: For those who spend fewer than six hours in bed
If you don't allow yourself enough time in bed (at least six hours), try the following:

Pick your wake-up time based on existing commitments (work, kids, carpool, family, and/or social commitments, etc.). Most of us know the time we *have* to get up, but we don't know when we should go to bed so our biological rhythms are aligned with physical (real) time. Take your wake-up time and work backward, factoring in sleep cycles, to learn what time you need to hit the hay. For example:

You wake at 6:30 A.M. (Most people wake by 7 A.M.)

You assume you need to have five sleep cycles. (Cycles will vary in length, but five is a conservative, reasonable number. If you're over the age of fifty-five, then consider four.)

You guess that your first cycle is a robust 100 minutes while the remaining cycles are ninety minutes. So here's how it goes:

$90 \times 4 = 360 + 100$ minutes $= 460$ minutes.

Subtract 460 minutes from your 6:30 A.M. wake time and you get 10:50 P.M.

Your bedtime is thus 10:30 P.M., giving you twenty minutes to fall asleep.

Experiment #2: For those who have a hard time falling or staying asleep

If you have a hard time falling or staying asleep, try the following:

Take a guess as to how much sleep (in hours) on average you get. Select your wake time and count the hours backward. For example:

You wake at 6:30 A.M. and you usually get 6.5 hours of sleep.

Your bedtime is around 11:30 P.M. if you're going to fall asleep by midnight. (Give yourself between twenty and thirty minutes to fall asleep.)

You may have noticed that the two previous exercises start with the same wake time but have different bedtimes. In Experiment #1 you are establishing your optimal sleep time (i.e., what you want to achieve), so if you are depriving yourself and don't feel alert the next day, lengthening your sleep will likely make you feel better. Remember, Experiment #1 is for those who fall asleep and stay asleep just fine but are very tired the next day. But in Experiment #2, you are now considering your actual sleep. If you have a mild form of insomnia, then getting into bed earlier may not be a great idea for you because you will lie there awake and very much alert to your wakefulness.

On average, about 55 percent of people are morning people, and 41 percent consider themselves evening people. Are you a lark or an owl?

Experiment #3

Are you early to bed and early to rise? Or are you a night owl?

In some cases I see people who force themselves to wake and sleep at certain times, especially if work and social activities dictate their schedules and boundaries. Letting your social, family, and work life run your sleep-wake schedule instead of the reverse—especially when these two factors compete—can be the root of many sleep problems. To compromise, find out what your body wants and then take that into consideration when trying to make some adjustments to both your sleep-wake schedule and the commitments you make during the day.

Review the list below to see which reflects you best:

	Early Bird	**Night Owl**
I feel alert:	in the early morning	late in the evening
I feel the most sleepy:	in the early evening	past 11 P.M.
I enjoy waking up:	6 A.M. or earlier	8 A.M. or later
I have the most energy:	a few hours after waking	the last hours before bed

For example, if you are a night owl who needs to be at work by 8:30, instead of getting up at 6:30 to get ready, try moving that time to 6:45 and then 7:00. A little time will make a big difference. Also, a quick tip: Never use the "snooze" button; all it does is allow you to go back into light, unrefreshing sleep, which does little good at the end of the night.

If you can't do this on your own, you might try light therapy. You can purchase or rent a light box (refer to Appendix B for resources) and reset your body's internal clock through exposure to light therapy at specific times. For example, if you have a tendency to be a night owl and sleep in too late, given your commitments, when you wake up, place a light box slightly above your line of vision and have it shine at least 5,000 lux of light for thirty to forty-five minutes each day. Over the course of a week you should be able to go to bed about thirty minutes earlier and wake thirty minutes earlier. The same holds true for moving the clock in the opposite direction. If you need to delay going to bed until a little later and get up a little later in the morning, you'd use the light exposure in the evenings. The Litebook Company makes a fantastic portable light box (www.litebook.com). You can also find other quality light boxes elsewhere. (By the way, bright light therapy has many uses, such as aiding in jet lag, seasonal blues, low mood, fatigue, and shift work issues. But it also has certain limitations. If you have a history of eye problems, including cataracts or macular degeneration, speak with your opthalmologist first before using one of these.) You can start by going to my Web site at www.soundsleepsolutions.com, where I'll direct you to reputable companies.

Once you have a good idea of how much sleep you need and when you need to get that sleep, regularize a sleep schedule and follow it consistently for seven consecutive days. The key here is to wake at the same time *every single day*, including weekends. So buy a good alarm clock, and tell your bed partner what time you need to be up. You may want to get two alarm clocks—one you use to alert you when it's time to get ready for bed, and one you use for your wake time. If you have a wristwatch that has a timer on it, use that to tell you "time to wind down and get ready for bed."

Remember: Sleep needs are individual; some people need nine hours, while others are energized after six.

Starting a Sleep Diary

Beginning with Night 1, you're going to start a sleep diary. Get a good notebook or journal in which you'll feel comfortable writing. We'll keep it simple at the start, and add more details to the record a bit later on. Here's what I want you to note this first week every morning upon waking (so keep this diary at your bedside):

- lights-out time
- how long you think it took you to fall asleep
- the time you woke up
- the quality of your sleep (rate 1–10 with 1 = poor, and 10 = great)
- how refreshed you feel in the A.M. (rate 1–10)

(Use the sample sleep diary in Appendix A to guide you.)

NIGHT 2: DEVELOP A BEDTIME ROUTINE

So how was your first night at your new bedtime? Were you tired to-day or well rested? If well rested or more rested, you are on your way! Great job. If you are more tired (and you usually experience insomnia) do not take a nap and stick to your schedule. It will work.

On this second day, you're still working on finding the optimal bed-time given your mandatory wake time and personal sleep cycles. In ad-dition to that task, I want you to establish a bedtime routine.

Myth Buster:
I can't turn my mind off! (This is the number one complaint people tell me who have insomnia or poor quality sleep.)
I think my sleep problems are caused by a chemical imbalance.
My poor sleep is ruining my life.
A nightcap helps me sleep.
The only way I can sleep is with medication.
The truth:
You *can* turn your mind off. One of the best ways is through distrac-tion, relaxation, and meditation. I'll give you some tips and tricks for this on the fifth night; you can overcome this.

Sleep problems are not typically caused by a chemical imbalance. Only in extremely rare and exceptional cases is poor sleep caused by a chemical im-balance. A simple blood test can identify some of these types of problems, such as a malfunctioning thyroid and hormonal (e.g., testosterone) issues.

Poor sleep does not have to ruin your life. I've treated hundreds of sleep-deprived people who believed there was no hope for them . . . and now they're sleeping dreamily.

A nightcap is not the answer to getting to sleep easily. An alcoholic drink can help you fall asleep quickly, but you'll wake up later on and have trouble returning to sleep. Too much alcohol too close to bedtime will also reduce the quality of your sleep.

Medication is not the only way to sound sleep. The main thrust of this book is non-pharmacological treatments for sleep. If you do require medication, that's not a big deal and it won't likely be forever.

Signaling to your body that "Hey, it's time to get ready for bed" is very important on both a conscious and a subconscious level. When you were a kid, you may have had parents who gave you a warm bath and then read to you as a signal for bedtime. It was easy, then, to get to sleep. As adults, we rarely take the time to perform bedtime habits that ultimately help us prepare for slumber and fall asleep quickly. Well, it's time to be a kid again.

Set aside an hour before bedtime during which you disengage from anything that is too stimulating. This is your "Power-Down Hour." Examples of things *you cannot do* during this hour include:

- *writing/receiving e-mail, surfing the Web, or playing computer games
- *listening to phone messages and returning calls
- paying bills
- watching TV (we'll discuss this more later)
- having important conversations with your spouse
- eating or drinking (except water)
- reading or referring to anything work related, such as newspaper articles, manuals, textbooks, PowerPoint presentations, and so on

During the first half hour, complete all of your mindless chores, such as walking the dog, feeding the animals, washing dishes or doing laundry, setting your alarm clock, locking the doors, etc. Set your house up for nighttime. Share these chores with your spouse and communicate other things that may need to get done, including tending to children's needs. Lightly share how the day went. If your spouse does not have the same time for bed as you do, then work out an arrangement that won't disturb the one who goes to bed first (the "first" spouse). This may entail having the "second" spouse enter the bedroom after the first one has fallen asleep, or having the second spouse already in the room when the first is going to sleep. If you have kids, you must decide upon shifts for who takes care of the kids and when (refer to Chapter 3).

Next, consider doing all of your hygiene activities: brushing your teeth, washing your face, taking nighttime medications, slipping into your loose-fitting bedclothes, and turning off all the lights in your bedroom,

*If checking e-mail or voice mail and returning messages is very stimulating for you, or it makes you extra worried and nervous to think you've got messages awaiting you, you may want to find a cutoff time for dealing with messages—no matter what time you go to bed. For example, you can make a rule of not checking or returning messages after 7 p.m. If the phone's ring bothers you psychologically, turn your ringer off after that time, too. Guard your "communicationless" hours of the night. Also let people know you will not receive messages during certain hours. Then they do not expect you to answer them, and you have less stress.

closets, and bathrooms except for the night-lights. If your spouse is going to be going to bed later, make sure that you have installed the proper night-lights so he or she can get to the bedroom and bathroom without having to turn on lights that will disturb you.

Dim the lights in your bedroom so there is only bedside and no overhead lighting. Be sure to close (and clip!) the shades.

Scheduling in sex before sleeping can be tricky. If sex is on the menu (which isn't always predictable!), you should back up your preparation time for bed, and if your response to sex is wakefulness, then you must be careful about how you include sex in your bedtime routine. You may find that you have to back up your winding-down time to about two hours prior to sleep. Experiment with the timing of sex and keep a record of how you feel the next day in your journal. For more on trying to coordinate two different types of sleepers with one need for sexual activity, refer to Chapter 6, where I cover sleep and sex.

Once you've readied the house and your bedroom for sleep, you should have about fifteen minutes left over (from that one hour). This is your relaxation and meditation time. On Night 5 we'll delve into describing several techniques to calm yourself in preparation for sleep. For now, I want you to try the following exercise, which you'll then rate the next morning, and try a new method tomorrow night. After several days of experimenting with different bedtime relaxation practices, you can pinpoint which ones really work well for you. I bet you'll find that more than one is helpful, which is great because I want you to have an arsenal of weapons to use at night for relaxation and sleeping.

Tonight (Night 2): Lie down in a comfortable spot (e.g., on your bed or on a nearby lounge chair or couch) and take time to reflect, say your prayers, or meditate. Your meditation can be quite simple; try clearing your mind by thinking of a field of pure white snow.

In the morning (on Day 3), you will complete your sleep diary's second entry. Describe which technique you used for relaxation and its effectiveness. Remember the information you need to record:

- lights-out time
- how long you think it took you to fall asleep
- the time you woke up

- the quality of your sleep (rate 1–10)
- how refreshed you feel in the A.M. (rate 1–10)
- On a scale of 1–10, how relaxed did self-reflection/meditation while lying down make you feel?

NIGHT 3: EVALUATE DAYTIME HABITS AND ROUTINES

> **Myth Buster:** *How I live out my day shouldn't affect how I sleep at night.* Quite the contrary, what you do—including what you eat and drink—from the moment you wake up to the time to you try to wind down for the night does affect the quality of your sleep.

How were nights one and two? Are you finding your sleep number? Are you getting closer? Keep trying. Rarely does someone find it until the end of the first week. By now you've learned a lot about how your daytime routines directly—and indirectly—affect your sleep habits. But if you haven't stopped to look critically at (and calculate) your daily doses of caffeine, alcohol, and/or nicotine, your challenge starts on Day 3. You're going to begin to monitor your consumptions and take actions as necessary.

Notes on Alcohol

Alcohol is metabolized relatively rapidly, at the rate of approximately one glass of wine or one-half pint of beer per hour (this is why you hear the "one drink per hour" rule). Therefore, if you were to drink four to five drinks in the three hours before bedtime, your alcohol concentrations in the blood would approach zero approximately two hours after you had fallen asleep. During the first part of the night, the alcohol tends to shorten the time it takes to go to sleep, increase non–rapid eye movement sleep (some of the lighter sleep), and reduce REM sleep. But as the withdrawal hits in the last half of the night, the result is shallow, disrupted sleep, increased REM sleep, increased dream or nightmare recall, and sympathetic arousal, including tachycardia and sweating. Sleep may also be interrupted by gastric irritation, headache, a full bladder, and a "rebound wakefulness." Your response to alcohol may not be the same as your sibling's or spouse's. For example, in some people the adverse effects of alcohol continue after blood alcohol concentrations are zero. Moderate drinking in the late afternoon—the so-called "happy hour"—may disrupt sleep during the last half of the night, long after alcohol has disappeared from the blood.

> Interestingly, no systematic scientific data exist, to our knowledge, about the effects of alcohol taken at low doses at bedtime on sleep in non-alcoholic, chronic insomniac patients who regularly use alcohol to promote sleep at night. We don't know if tolerance has developed to the side effects or the soporific benefits (sleepiness feelings) of alcohol. In other words, no one knows whether a "nightcap" is helpful or harmful in individuals who imbibe every night.

The Rules on Alcohol if You Drink

1. Take a multivitamin with minerals that morning. This is to replace what you will likely sweat out.

2. Consume at least forty ounces of water the day prior to drinking. This again helps prevent dehydration.

3. Drink one glass of water with each drink and don't start another without finishing your glass of water.

4. Go for clear liquids and white wines (these have less of a likelihood of hangover). Avoid sugary blends, such as cocktail mixers/syrups and regular soda.

5. Remember to go to bed at a reasonable time (preferably your usual time) so you're not increasing sleep deprivation while drinking (the double whammy).

Notes on Nicotine

It's easy to forget that nicotine is a stimulant when so many smokers claim to "have a smoke" to relax themselves. One of the most perpetuated myths about nicotine is that it acts as a sedative and has a calming effect. Nicotine can stay in the body for as long as fourteen hours. The effects of smoke on sleep depend largely on an individual's smoking habits (how much he or she smokes), but in general, nicotine reduces total sleep time and REM sleep time. It's also been shown to worsen sleep-disordered breathing. Having said that, however, smokers who experience cravings due to nicotine-withdrawal symptoms in the middle of the night can be rudely awakened by the need to smoke and, once they do, they can then go back to sleep. (In fact, insomnia is among a smoker's most common complaints.) It's, therefore, a mixed bag of issues when it comes to those addictive drags.

Although the benefits to quitting smoking are obvious to most of us by now, I'm not going to suggest you eliminate smoking entirely from your life in pursuit of sound sleep. Why not? If I told you the only way to sound sleep was through quitting smoking forever, you'd probably put this book down. Instead, I'm going to give you permission to continue smoking (hoping you do achieve a smoke-free life at some point) and tell you how to work around your smoking habits so you can achieve better sleep. This actually can act as a control because if your sleep does not improve after completing this month's program, at least you'll know that smoking is probably having a greater impact on your ability to sleep well than you currently accept. It may be the only thing that's keeping you from getting a good night's sleep. Then your next goal will be to quit (which is another book).

The Rules on Nicotine if You Smoke

1. Don't stop smoking during the program; continue smoking as you would normally. Trying to do two things at once will be too difficult.

2. Try having your last cigarette of the night about one hour earlier than normal. Keep yourself busy with your nighttime routine and get to bed on time.

3. If you experience withdrawal while doing this program and you wake up in the middle of the night craving a cigarette, you are moving too fast. Have your last cigarette just thirty minutes earlier than normal.

4. Consider chewing nicotine gum or using the patch so your body does not go through withdrawal and wake you. But be careful because both the patch and gum have been known to increase the likelihood of poor sleep.

Notes on Caffeine

If you've already tried the Action Plan outlined in Chapter 2 for the caffeine junkie, stay on that plan. If you haven't, now is when you can go back to that chapter and incorporate those recommendations here on Day 3. But if those tips don't completely solve your problems, or if you want to take it a step further, it's time to be stricter with your caffeine cutoff point—the time at which you no longer consume any-thing that contains caffeine for the rest of the day.

The Rules on Caffeine if You Simply Have to Have It

1. Stop drinking highly caffeinated beverages by 2 P.M., and move over to less caffeinated drinks. For example, get all of your drip coffee and espresso-based drinks in you as soon as you can (preferably before noon). Then, once the afternoon hits, go for diluted teas and soft drinks. Watch what you're consuming, however; some teas and soft drinks (energy and sports drinks, too) can contain a sneaky amount of caffeine, so pay atten-tion. Because many beverages sold today don't show caffeine content on their labels, gaining experience with how they affect you is a must. The goal is to be drinking non-caffeinated beverages after 5 P.M., such as juices and herbal teas. (If you can skip decaf coffee altogether, that'd be best.)

2. Evaluate your sleep each morning from 1 (poor) to 10 (great) based on this caffeine cutoff time and record how you feel. Did you wake up with a headache in the middle of the night or the next morn-ing? (This could indicate caffeine-withdrawal symptoms.) Was it easier to fall asleep? If you rate your sleep at a 5 or less, back up that cutoff time to 4 P.M. and repeat the exercise.

3. If a 4 P.M. cutoff time still gets you to rank your sleep at a 5 or less, wait two days and then back up your cutoff time to 3 P.M. Remember: You are looking for a balance here between your sleep and withdrawal. You may end up staying at the same place for your caffeine cutoff for over a week if needed.

4. If you just must have a pick-me-up late in the day and a cup of joe sounds like the only thing that can save you, try your best to reach for a less potent alternative like green or black tea diluted well with water. Sometimes a drink of cold sparkling water can liven you up just as well as that cup of joe (especially since sleepiness can be a sign of dehydra-tion). And I've heard some people swear that having an apple can im-part some energy without any caffeine whatsoever.

Diet and exercise can also impact your sleep, but we'll get to those notes and rules a bit later on.

Today's relaxation technique: Make a list of the biggest stressors of your day, along with a plan to deal with them. This acts as "closure" to the day. If you cannot find a solution to any of these, write "will take care of tomorrow" and remove it from your mind.

> If you've succeeded in switching to less potent caffeine drinks such as tea and you want to take it further, recycle your tea bags later in the day. That is, hold on to that tea bag that made a strong cup in the morning, and make another cup of tea with the same bag in the afternoon for a boost. The second time around will still have the taste of tea, but contain much less caffeine. Another option is to discard the first cup of tea made from a fresh tea bag, and make another cup. Also, don't squeeze the tea out of the tea bag, as these drops of tea contain more caffeine. To avoid caffeine entirely, try grain-based hot beverages and caffeine-free herbal teas as alternatives to coffee and tea.

What to record in your diary at the start of Day 4:
- lights-out time
- how long you think it took you to fall asleep
- the time you woke up
- the quality of your sleep (rate 1–10)
- how refreshed you feel in the A.M. (rate 1–10)
- On a scale of 1–10 how relaxed did listing out your stressors and their solutions make you feel?
- How much:
  - ➤ caffeine you ingested and when
  - ➤ nicotine you ingested and when
  - ➤ alcohol you ingested and when

NIGHT 4: CHECK ON THE BEDROOM ENVIRONMENT

> **Myth Buster:** *It takes too much money and time to make—literally— the bedroom of my dreams.* Your bedroom doesn't have to cost a fortune to create. Start by focusing on the simplest modifications, such as the placement of furniture and replacing certain lightbulbs with lower wattage. You don't have to spend a fortune making it look suitable for *Architectural Digest*. You just have to make it perfect for one thing only: inviting sleep to scamper in regularly each and every night.

In Chapter 4 we took a tour of creating the ideal bedroom environment. Don't let the To Dos of that chapter overwhelm you; go step-by-step and work toward building the bedroom of your dreams over time. Obviously you're probably not going to start painting your room or calling the best interior decorator in town for a consult today. I just want you to keep thinking of simple ways to spruce up the quality of your bedroom environment easily and quickly. You may even want to list out "long-term goals" and "short-term goals" for making your bedroom a true sanctuary for sleep in the coming year. For example, write down in your diary "shop for and buy a new mattress" under long-term goal. Write down "buy night-lights for all hallways and bathrooms" under short-term goals.

Here, on Day 4, I want you to review your bedroom setup and see what you can do next to add to that makeover. Don't know where to start? The following twenty-three steps will help you take action right away without costing you much time, effort, or money. These are the most important things to consider purchasing and/or doing as soon as possible:

1. Clean your bedroom and make sure you have a clear path to the bed, bathroom, and out the door.

2. Replace all bulbs to 40 watts, or have dimmers installed on light switches or for bedside lamps.

3. If needed, purchase eye shades that don't allow your eyelashes to rub against them. Consider ones with built-in aromatherapy.

4. Test your mattress. If it hasn't been turned (rotated if it's a pillow-top mattress) in a year, do it now. If it's older than seven years, it's time to buy a new one.

5. Remove all possible allergens in the room, and address the sources of such allergens such as laundry detergent, pillow fillings, and pets.

6. Get rid of dust ruffles.

7. Install night-lights to lead you to the bathroom without having to turn on the lights.

8. Purchase a sound-dampening device, such as earplugs, a noise machine, or a fan.

9. Ensure the temperature is between sixty-five and seventy degrees Fahrenheit. You might sleep better when the temperature is on the high side during the winter and on the cool side during the summer.

10. Buy a humidifier for winter (when you turn the heat on) and sum-

mer if you live in a dry climate. Maintain air freshness. Have your air ducts cleaned, and open windows during the day to allow fresh air to circulate.

11. Test your pillows; if they don't spring back when folded, replace them. (Refer to the Pic-a-Pillow guidelines on page 108.)

12. Consider new sheets, but don't be fooled by the expensive thread count.

13. Buy some aromatherapy. (I have multiple suggestions on my Web site.)

14. If you have a television in your room, buy a timer for it if you don't already have one installed, or at least learn how to use the one you have. You want this because as the volume changes from show to show and commercial to commercial, it can bring you to lighter sleep throughout the night. Use earphones if you are going to watch TV while your bed partner sleeps.

15. Buy a book light if you (or your bed partner) need it.

16. Move your bed so that is does not face east.

17. Make sure your drapes allow for total darkness.

18. Remove visually distracting decorations or wall adornments and replace them with only peaceful items that are instantly calming to the eye.

19. Buy a few sets of new bedclothes. Do not sleep in underwear that you have worn all day long. Make sure you have a set that will keep you warm in the winter and a set that will keep you cool in the summer. When you put your bedtime clothes on, let this be a signal for you to disengage from the day and avoid further chores and work. Let your clothes tell you it's almost time to sleep.

20. Consider over-the-counter nasal decongestants that you know work well for you (or your bed partner) to avoid one possible factor in snoring. Watch out for decongestants, however, that contain stimulating ingredients like pseudoephedrine.

21. Buy herbal tea (non-caffeinated).

22. Buy a good multivitamin with extra iron.

23. If you suffer from acid reflux or GERD, raising the head of your bed between six and eight inches will help keep stomach acid from flowing into your esophagus while you are sleeping. You can do this by putting blocks underneath your bed frame or by placing a foam wedge under the head of your mattress. (Using extra pillows will not work.)

24. Download my relaxation MP3 (if you haven't already)—it's free; www.soundsleepsolutions.com.

Refer to Chapter 4 for further details (see checklist for a quick review). Make an effort to set some goals for how you're going to complete the perfect bedroom over time using the diary in Appendix A.

The Bedroom Checklist—at a Glance

The following are the main topics covered in Chapter 4. Go through this list to ensure you've considered all these important factors in creating the ideal sleep environment.

- ❏ furniture arrangement and special layout (away from direct sunlight or nearby noise?)
- ❏ wall colors, paint or paper (mood—calm and peaceful?)
- ❏ wall hangings and adornments (mood—calm and peaceful?)
- ❏ quality of mattress (good?)
- ❏ bedding linens (clean, soft, and comfortable?)
- ❏ pillows, blankets, covers (allergen-free, comfortable?)
- ❏ source and intensity of light (natural and artificial, including monitors)
- ❏ source and intensity of sound (natural and artificial, including TV)
- ❏ odors (pleasant?)
- ❏ air quality (good?)
- ❏ temperature and humidity (around seventy degrees Fahrenheit and 65 percent humidity?)

Ask yourself: How does your bedroom make you *feel* when you enter it? If feelings of frustration from endless nights of sleeplessness wash over you, now's the time to start turning that around. Once you start changing physical elements to your bedroom, you can then begin to change the deeper, more psychological elements that influence your sleep.

Today's relaxation technique: Read something light and fun, or really boring (avoid any stimulating material, such as a page-turning book that will keep you up or an intense article that will get you thinking too hard).

What to record in your diary at the start of Day 5:
- lights-out time
- how long you think it took you to fall asleep
- the time you woke up
- the quality of your sleep (rate 1–10)
- how refreshed you feel in the A.M. (rate 1–10)
- On a scale of 1–10, how relaxed did reading something light/ fun/boring make you feel?
- How much:
  - ➤ caffeine you ingested and when
  - ➤ nicotine you ingested and when
  - ➤ alcohol you ingested and when
  - ➤ What's left to do to your room to make it a better sleep environment?

NIGHT 5: PREPARE YOUR BODY FOR BED WITH STRETCHING AND RELAXATION

Myth Buster: *Relaxation techniques work for everybody.* This isn't necessarily true. Everyone is different when it comes to unwinding and preparing for bed. You have to experiment with an assortment of techniques to determine which works best for you.

Today I want you to look back in your diary and take an average of Nights 2 through 4 for sleep quality and how refreshed you felt in the mornings. These numbers will correspond to your level of relaxation once you begin to learn these techniques on Night 5.

There are as many different relaxation and meditation techniques as there are personalities. So-called high-strung people—those who don't appear to relax easily and who live in "hypermetabolic" states in which their body is producing more adrenaline than usual—usually need a different set of techniques from people who are typically laid-back and relaxed all the time. Excuse the stereotype, but think of a frenetic, fast-talking and speed-walking stockbroker on the floors of Wall Street versus a novelist who isn't psychologically chained to a stock ticker all day. Do you think these two types of people can share the same relaxation techniques? Maybe, but maybe not. In fact, one may respond very well to a certain set of techniques while the other doesn't. For example, one may need a vacation from mental activities while the other needs to loosen up tense muscles. And these can come from two different relaxation techniques.

Unfortunately, there is no one-size-fits-all practice that I can teach you and that will be guaranteed to work for you every night. Not everyone can relax easily, and not everyone responds the same to a particular method of relaxation. Furthermore, a relaxation technique can work well for you for a while and then be less effective over time. People seem to grow in and out of them with age and circumstance. If you've been a student of any martial arts, yoga, or other practice that includes some meditative skills and you know what works for you, then it will be easier for you to draw from your own experience. But if you've never meditated or learned any relaxation skills, then this will be a new challenge for you. Whether you need to acquire physical, mental, and/or emotional relaxation skills, understand that all such skills require practice, time, and effort. They must be learned and then used over and over again as you develop them further.

Let's begin to experiment with a few relaxation techniques here on Night 5. Record which ones you choose and how they make you feel in your diary. If you find that none of these help you at all, and they make you frustrated or even antsy, don't feel pressure to do them. You just might be the type who's relaxed enough as it is. In fact, forcing yourself to perform relaxation techniques can actually disrupt your sleep.

As an aside, if you discover that, as you stretch out your body and relax your muscles you have lots of tension, aches, or pains that aren't being helped by the stretching, go back into the bathroom and draw yourself a moderately hot bath. Your journey to the bathroom should still be under dim light (you should have a night-light installed in hallways and bathrooms). Be sure to pour in some aromatherapy. Make sure that you schedule this bath in at the start of the hour the next day, however. It's best to have a bath about an hour before you actually get into bed.

Below are instructions to a few techniques you can try. All of these can be done on the bed. Start by **picking one or two** for today and then try another combination of two tomorrow. See which ones put you at most ease. Choose a different combination each day and see if you can come up with a winning set of exercises that you can do whenever you want to take a time-out and put your mind and body to rest. They should only take about ten to fifteen minutes to do. If you awaken in the middle of the night feeling tense and stressed, you can do one and then go back to bed. You might find it helpful to read and practice these poses and stretches during the day so you can learn them by memory before trying to perform them at bedtime. Or, record their instructions so you can listen to them with a headset.

It's also important to check in with your doctor if you have any medical or physical issues that should be addressed in light of doing these exercises. Be mindful of your own limitations and individual conditions, whether you're starting an exercise program or simply commencing a nighttime stretching and/or yoga routine.

Relaxed Standing Forward Bend. Stand with your legs wide apart (aligned with hips) and slightly bent. Bend over at your waist and let your arms extend toward the floor, shaking them out if you wish. Let your head hang as your arms remain dangling. Release all the tension in your neck and shoulders and sway from side to side. Feel the weight of your body as you hang loosely and try to continue releasing all tension in your body.

The Point-to-Point Release (NOTE: The following exercise is outlined on a track you can download for free at www.sounsleepsolutions.com. Progressive relaxation exercises like this one are easiest to do while listening to the instructions.)

Lie on your back in the relaxation pose (see box, page 197). Close your eyes, and systematically address every part of your body, sensing each part's weight and letting everything sink into the bed. Start at your head and move toward your toes. Begin by softening your forehead, eyes, face, and jaw. Tensing and then releasing each muscle group will help tight muscles loosen, especially those in the neck and shoulders. Continue giving attention to each area of your body—the arms, the trunk, and the legs—until you reach your toes. Surrender to gravity.

Stay in this relaxed state for a few minutes, letting the bed support you. Focus on your breathing, releasing all other concerns. You may also want to include some guided imagery here (see page 198). Let your breath come from deep in your abdomen, and let it flow smoothly, slowly, and evenly. This simple exercise is a way of telling your mind and body that it's okay to stop thinking, working, and struggling.

Cobbler's Pose with Head Rolls. Sit straight and tall on the bed with the soles of the feet together and the heels close to the pelvis (use a pillow, if necessary, to avoid rounding the lower back). Clasp your hands around the ankles, relaxing the knees down. Lift the lower back and extend upward through the whole spine. Lift your chest, extending through the neck and crown of the head. Now focus on your breath as you release resistance and get comfortable in the pose. Drop your chin to your chest. Release all tension in your neck, feeling the weight of your head. Begin to roll to the left and turn your chin toward your shoulder, keeping your neck relaxed. Return your head to the center of your chest and repeat the roll over to your right shoulder. Then raise you head up again and tilt it gently to the left, then to the right. Make sure your shoulders remain down and relaxed, tilting your head toward each of them in sequential moves.

Deep Breathing. One of the easiest ways to relax is to simply focus on breathing and take in long, deep, abdominal breaths. This means you let everything else relax itself and you concentrate solely on inhaling all the way in so your lungs fill with air and your belly extends outward. Then, you exhale slowly and squeeze everything out of your lungs. Here's how to do this step-by-step:

- Lie on your back.
- Slowly relax your body (point-to-point, as described in the text).
- Begin to inhale slowly through your nose if possible. Feel that air filling up from the bottom of your chest cavity upward. Be sure to do this slowly, over eight to ten seconds.
- Hold your breath for a second or two.
- Then quietly and easily relax and let the air out. Squeeze everything out of your lungs.
- Wait a few seconds and repeat this cycle.
- You can continue this breathing technique for as long as you like until you fall asleep.

The Cat Stretch. Rest on your hands and knees, with your palms directly under your shoulders and your knees directly under your hips (this is called the table pose). While exhaling and squeezing out every bit of air on your lungs, contract the abdominal muscles, tuck the pelvis, and round the spine, arching the back upward—like a cat on a fence. Then, while inhaling, release the abdominal muscles completely as you lift your sitting bones, spread the buttocks, lift the head, and arch your spine down. Keep the arms straight and the weight evenly distributed between the hands and knees. Repeat these two movements about five times.

> **The Relaxation Pose ("Savasana," in yoga-speak; or, better yet, the "Corpse Pose").** This pose is usually done on a firm, flat surface with a thick cushion to support the neck and head. If you wish, you can try this on the floor beside your bed or on the bed itself. You might find, however, that for some exercises, this pose is best done on a firmer surface. Lie on your back and close your eyes. Lift and lengthen the back of your neck until it feels comfortable. Relax and lengthen your spine without bending to either side. Rest your legs about twelve to fourteen inches apart. Rest your arms six to eight inches from the sides, palms turned upward (they may, however, roll inward). Bring the shoulder blades slightly together, and draw them down toward your waist, opening the chest.

The Sponge. This can be done lying down (in the Relaxation Pose), standing or sitting; it's a combination of deep breathing with some imagery. Once you've gotten into your most relaxed state, imagine you're a sponge, lying in a pool of warm water. Imagine the water extending forever in all directions around you. Feel the warmth bathing your skin. The pores of your body are like the pores of the sponge. As you breathe in, you are drawing in this warm, relaxing water through every pore of your body. Feel the warmth penetrating your skin.

As you breathe out, the water is soaking into your body, filling you up. Feel the water seeping into all the corners of your body, penetrating your muscles, soaking into your organs, bathing every cell in warmth. Focus on feelings of heaviness and warmth.

Next time you breathe in, imagine you are drawing in the water through your pores.

Each time you breathe out, feel the water soaking into your body, filling all the corners. As the water soaks into every part of you, it feels peaceful. And you feel heavier, sinking into the water.

GUIDED IMAGERY AND MIND GAMES

The Sponge is a good example of using guided imagery to relax and stretch deeper into oneself. Visualization can be a handy tool for detaching the mind from the day and falling asleep quickly. Playing mind games that won't rev up the brain and stimulate you can also be quite helpful. Below are some more examples of exercises you can do to mindlessly "think" your way to sleep; some entail your imagination, others get you to think a certain way. The goal is to let sleep sneak up on you and take over without you paying much attention because you're thinking about something boring, imaginary, or performing a monotonous task in your brain.

Choose one of these to try tonight after one or two stretches. Choose another one tomorrow, and so on.

- Count backward from 1,000 in groups of seven (i.e., count every seventh number from 1,000). This isn't easy.
- Imagine being an astronaut on a space walk. You're floating around the world, watching Earth rotate as you weightlessly move around it. Or, imagine floating on a cloud or out at sea on a wave.
- Imagine that your thoughts are bubbles and let them float up through your mind to the surface of your head and then . . . poof! . . . they disappear out of your head.
- Picture your favorite, most relaxing place to be. The place may be on a sunny beach with the warm ocean breezes caressing you, swinging in a hammock in the mountains or on a desert island. Visualize yourself in that peaceful setting. See and feel your surroundings, hear the peaceful sounds, smell the flowers or the salty air.
- Imagine falling deep into a vortex, and the deeper you go, the closer you are to sleep. You may find it helpful to think about riding down an elevator, or sinking deeper and deeper into the bed to the point where you can't tell where your body ends and the bed begins. As you go farther and farther into this vortex, your breathing becomes deeper, your body becomes weightless, and your mind loses focus. You are approaching sleep.

- If your thoughts won't let your mind stop, picture yourself standing in front of a chalkboard. See yourself writing down all those thoughts onto the board. Now step up to the board and erase them all. Now admire the clean, blank board. Continue to stare at it and try to keep your mind totally blank while doing so.
- Describe your home village, town, or city in the greatest possible detail, as though to a complete stranger.
- Work your way through the alphabet from A to Z and come up with four- or five-letter words beginning with each letter.
- Spell long words.
- Recite a song, poem, or anthem, such as the Pledge of Allegiance, and then try to do it backward.

THE SUN SALUTES IN THE MORNING:
IT'S NOT JUST ABOUT THE NIGHT

A great stretch to start your day is to perform the Sun Salute, which is one of the most basic sequences of yoga poses. As its name implies, you are greeting the new day by saluting the sun, but you don't have to actually be facing the sun or looking at it. It may even be raining or snowing outside and you can still perform your sun salutations. (Warning: Discuss any physical limitations you might have with your doctor. Consult with your doctor before starting any physical program.)

Sun Salutes are often performed in sets of five, but if you are new to the practice, begin with two or three. Each time you flow through this sequence, synchronize your breath with the movements of your body.

This exercise will help awaken your body, mind, and spirit first thing in the morning. It stretches muscles and activates your mind. In this exercise, you will inhale when your body is open and exhale when your body is folding closed. For further instruction on how these moves flow, go to my Web site at www.soundsleepsolutions.com. Here's the gist of how it works (as soon as you roll out of bed, find a space close by to do this):

1. Stand tall in a straight column. Your feet should be together, the bases of your big toes touching and your heels slightly apart. Distribute your weight evenly over both feet. Take a few deep breaths, then establish a slow, steady rhythm for your breath.

On an exhale, bring the palms of your hands together in front of your chest as if you're praying.

2. Next, inhale and stretch your arms out to the side and overhead, converging them together over your head as you bring your palms together again. Spread your shoulder blades and flex slightly back from the waist, hips forward. As you take your head back, gaze up at your thumbs. This is sending your greeting to the sun.

3. Exhale and bend forward, folding yourself *at the hips.* Place your hands beside your feet, bending at the knees slightly if you need to. Keep your arms strong; don't let yourself dangle loosely.

4. Inhale and lengthen your spine forward so that your back is flat, as if someone can now come rest a glass on top of it like a table. In this pose, lift your gaze so you're looking forward, and keep extending your spine. Your fingertips can stay on the floor or come up to the shins.

5. Inhale. Take the left leg back, touching the floor with your left knee and left toes. Your hands and right leg are still in front. Arch your back, lift your chin, and look up.

6. Now take the right leg back as you lift your left knee off the floor. Straighten your legs, supporting your body weight on your hands and toes. (This is called the Plank Pose.) In this pose, your arms are perpendicular to the floor, your shoulders are directly over the wrists, and your torso is parallel to the floor. Your palms should be flat on the floor, shoulder-distance apart, and your feet should be at hip distance. (You might feel like you're about to do some push-ups.) Take a full breath in as you lengthen through your spine.

7. As you exhale, lower your knees to the floor. Bend your arms at the elbows to lower your torso. Let your chest, then your forehead, touch the floor. Your hands should still be flat on the floor.

8. Inhale while lowering your hips to the floor. Arch your spine back. Look up, taking your head back. Pull your shoulders back and open your collarbones. Engage your legs, but relax your gluteal muscles.

9. Exhale and roll your weight over your toes and onto your feet, raising the hips up and back. Push your heels down and hang your head. (This is moving into the downward-facing Dog Pose.)* In this pose, you press the fingers and the palms into the floor. Your arms are straight, helping you press the hips up and back, keeping the spine straight and long. Your feet are hips' width apart with the toes facing

forward. Press the heels into the floor feeling a stretch in the back of the legs. The legs are straight, or you can have a small bend at the knees to keep the back flat. Let your head and neck hang freely from the shoulders or look up at the belly button. Remain here for five deep, long breaths.

10. On your fifth exhale, bend your knees and look between your hands. Then inhale and step or lightly hop your feet between your hands, returning to a standing forward bend.

11. Roll up your upper body and repeat the sequence.

*For step-by-step instruction with photos, go to my Web site, www.soundsleep solutions.com.

Action Reminder

Pick two of the stretches outlined on pages 195–201 to perform at the end of your bedtime routine. Then complete a deep-breathing exercise with some guided imagery. If you are not asleep within about twenty minutes, use the following mind game: Count backward from 1,000 in groups of seven (1,000 . . . 993 . . . 986 . . . 979 . . . 972 . . .).

What to record in your diary at the start of Day 6:
- lights-out time
- how long you think it took you to fall asleep
- the time you woke up
- the quality of your sleep (rate 1–10)
- how refreshed you feel in the A.M. (rate 1–10)
- On a scale of 1–10 how relaxed did your bedtime technique make you feel? Which stretches and/or guided imagery ideas did you try?
- How much:
  ➤ caffeine you ingested and when
  ➤ nicotine you ingested and when
  ➤ alcohol you ingested and when
  ➤ What's left to do to your room to make it a better sleep environment?
  ➤ Did you remember to do some stretching, such as the Sun Salute, in the morning?

NIGHT 6: FOCUS ON FOODS

Myth Buster: *Turkey will put you to sleep because of the enzymes it contains, which promote sleep.*

Sleep-friendly foods, such as turkey, may help you relax and fall asleep, but don't view them as "sleeping pills." You'd have to eat about forty pounds of turkey to get enough of that enzyme to make you sleepy. That enzyme is called tryptophan, which is an essential amino acid you must get from your diet to build certain proteins. This amino acid can also be found in chicken, pork, and cheese. But for it alone to be an effective sleeping agent, you'd also need to take it on an empty stomach, so consuming forty pounds of food for the purpose of the enzyme is counteractive. Tryptophan can, however, help regulate sleep in supplement form.

Diet has an impact in all that we do, from how we feel and how much energy we have (or don't have), to how well we sleep and whether we can even get to sleep on time at night. In general, a diet low in essential vitamins, minerals, and nutrients, for example, is likely to dampen the quality of your life both when you're awake and while you're sleeping, from a physical and psychological standpoint. Enough scientific evidence exists to support the connection between maintaining healthy eating habits and sleeping well. I won't be going into the details of what constitutes a healthy diet; there are plenty of other books and resources for that (start by referring to the American Heart Association, the American Cancer Society, or the Surgeon General, all of whose recommendations you can access online). Here, I'm going to concentrate on other issues related to food and sleep, and give you some pointers for making these two life-sustaining activities (eating and sleeping) work in synergy.

Keep in mind that everyone's rate of metabolism (and digestion) will differ slightly. Common sense says it's not wise to eat a heavy meal (one that's rich, fatty, and calorie-laden) just before bedtime. But some people who have a super-fast metabolism might be okay with such a meal within two hours of hitting the hay. Like so many other aspects to sound sleep, you have to pay attention to your body and experiment a little to find your own inner balance. None of these rules here are hard and fast.

One consequence to sleep is our metabolism slows down, which can have a big effect on what our bodies are still trying to digest within a few hours before bed. Not all foods pass through the stomach and down to the lower intestines at the same rate. The fluidity of your stomach's gastric juices also determines how long it takes to digest your food. Liquids, for example, usually pass through the stomach quite rapidly, but solids remain until they are well mixed. Fatty foods may remain in the stomach for three to six hours; foods high in protein tend to move through more quickly; and carbohydrates usually pass through more rapidly than either fats or proteins.

A heavy or very large meal might make you feel sleepy and lethargic, but because your digestive system has to work so hard to process all that food, it can keep you awake during the night. Feasting on a big meal asks your circulatory system to move more blood to your digestive tract. It asks your stomach to secrete more gastric acid. It asks your pancreas to become more active and produce digestive enzymes. It asks the smooth muscles around your intestines to become active. Basically, a large meal does anything but relax you. In addition, your digestive tracts are set up to work best when you are standing; lying down results in gravity pulling the "wrong way" to help food digest. Even though the practice of napping after a meal is common, it isn't ideal from the standpoint of digestion. Sitting and resting are fine. For example, enjoying one another's company around the table after a delicious meal is a good idea. But lying down to sleep just doesn't help digestion.

I also don't recommend increasing your intake of foods high in tryptophan (e.g., turkey) as a way of improving your sleep. Studies of tryptophan's impact on sleep have found only one phase of sleep—the first one when you're falling asleep—that's enhanced by tryptophan in supplemental form. Other aspects of sleep, such as the amount of deep sleep reached during the night, are actually harmed by supplemental tryptophan. As mentioned in the Myth Buster, it's better to regard tryptophan as a sleep regulator than a sleep inducer. You also don't want to go to bed hungry; otherwise hunger pangs can keep you up, too.

Here are some practical recommendations, many of which you've heard of because they constitute a healthy approach to food and diet:

- Make breakfast the largest meal of the day. Avoid high-sugar cereals or high-fat breakfast concoctions and load up instead on whole grains (oatmeal, high-fiber/low-sugar cereals) and get some protein into your A.M. routine as well. Don't forget to include a good source of vitamins and minerals, even if that comes from a pill or a drink.

- Lunch should be either a sandwich or a salad with some type of protein to help you work through the afternoon blahs. (A lunch too high in carbohydrates will only exacerbate your sleepiness.)
- Dinner needs to incorporate some protein but be on the complex carbohydrate track. This is when the timing of the meal is most important. It's best to schedule in your dinner about four hours prior to your self-prescribed bedtime. Why? This gives you plenty of time to metabolize whatever you've eaten that day. You may need to sneak in a snack closer to bedtime (about an hour prior), however, if you experience hunger pangs at night. That snack should be from the complex carbohydrate category, like a piece of whole grain toast with a thin spread of unprocessed peanut butter or a slice of cheese on top. The best bedtime snack is one that has both complex carbohydrates and a little protein, plus some calcium. Calcium helps the brain use the tryptophan to manufacture melatonin. This explains why dairy products, which contain both tryptophan and calcium, are one of the top sleep-inducing foods. And by combining carbohydrates together with a small amount of protein, your brain produces serotonin, which is known as the "calming hormone."

A high-carbohydrate meal stimulates the release of insulin, which helps clear from the bloodstream those amino acids that compete with tryptophan, thus allowing more of this natural sleep-inducing amino acid to enter the brain and manufacture sleep-inducing substances, such as serotonin and melatonin. Eating a high-protein meal without accompanying carbohydrates may keep you awake, since protein-rich foods also contain the amino acid tyrosine, which perks up the brain.

- Avoid heavily spiced foods or garlicky foods at dinner.
- Also avoid drinking too much of anything, water included, once you've finished your meal. It takes about ninety minutes for the body to process liquids, so with the exception of herbal tea during your prep time for sleep, limit liquids for at least ninety

minutes prior to bedtime. Otherwise, you'll need to urinate during the night, waking you up.

Best Dinners for Sleep

Meals that are high in carbohydrates and low to medium in protein will help you relax in the evening and set you up for a good night's sleep. Some ideas are:

- pasta with Parmesan cheese (you may want to avoid red, tomato-based sauces since the high acidity can increase the likelihood for reflux)
- scrambled eggs and cheese
- tofu stir-fry with brown rice
- hummus with whole wheat pita bread
- seafood
- meats and poultry with veggies (especially broccoli, spinach, and artichokes)
- tuna salad sandwich
- chili with beans (not spicy), and with a sweet potato
- sesame seeds (rich in tryptophan—for regulating sleep) sprinkled on salad with tuna chunks, and whole wheat crackers

Best Bedtime Snacks

Foods that are high in carbohydrates and calcium and are medium to low in protein also make ideal sleep-inducing bedtime snacks. Some examples are:

- apple pie and ice cream (my favorite but I don't indulge in this every night!)
- New York–style cheesecake
- whole-grain cereal with skim milk (steer clear of the high-sugar cereals)
- hazelnuts and tofu
- oatmeal and raisin cookies, and a glass of milk
- peanut butter sandwich
- fruit and sour cream or cottage cheese
- whole grain toast topped with one small slice of low-fat cheese
- whole wheat crackers topped with mild cheese
- a banana with one teaspoon of peanut butter

Bedtime snacks should be consumed about an hour before your actual bedtime, and should be within 200 calories—not more. It takes about an hour for the tryptophan in the foods to reach your brain, so don't wait until right before you hop into bed to have your snack.

Warning: If you are lactose intolerant you should use lactose-free products.

Kitchen Roundup

You learned in Chapter 5 how sleep affects your digestive hormones, and that some of the most wicked ingredients for maintaining a healthy diet are commonly found in all sorts of foods and beverages today. High fructose corn syrup, for example, can be in places you'd least expect it, like fat-free snacks and sodas, condiments, "lite" salad dressings, and low-fat ice cream. Trans fats also add danger to a lot of popular foods. I urge you to take a good look at what fills your refrigerator and kitchen cabinets. See if you can discard any products that contain trans fats and/or high fructose corn syrup. If you can't get rid of all such products, at least take note of where these ingredients lurk so you can be aware of them when you consume them.

Below is a list of foods you should definitely have in your kitchen when the season calls for them. I've also included a list of foods that you can have during the day but should avoid at dinner.

Keepers

milk, eggs, non-aged cheese
soy products
tuna, halibut
pumpkin, artichokes, avocados
almonds, walnuts
bok choy, asparagus, leafy greens, legumes
apricots, peaches, bananas, apples
oats, buckwheat, non-sugar cereals
potatoes

Losers at Dinner

heavy spices
tomato sauce/tomato-based foods like spaghetti sauce and pizza
drinks with carbonation

citrus fruits
chocolate
fatty and fried foods
garlic and onions
mint-flavored foods
spicy foods
anything with caffeine, such as coffee ice cream

Vitamins and Minerals: The Building Blocks for a Good Night's Rest

The body's need for vitamins and minerals increases enormously under certain conditions, and when essential vitamins and minerals are not readily available for everyday functions, your body wears down. A broken-down body is one that invites other health problems, the least of which is poor sleep. It's no surprise that one of the first consequences to vitamin and mineral deficiency is poor sleep or the inability to sleep at all. Let's look at some of the most important sleep-friendly vitamins and minerals to have ample supply of:

The Busy Bs: The B vitamins can help regulate the body's use of tryptophan and other amino acids. Because stress, smoking, alcohol, and environmental factors can quickly reduce the B vitamins in your system, sometimes it's not enough to rely on diet alone for a sufficient supply.

Vitamin B_3 (also called niacin) has been found to increase the effectiveness of tryptophan. Some studies suggest B_3 lengthens REM sleep and decreases the times an insomniac is awake during the night. What's more, Vitamin B_3 has been used to treat depression, which can be a big factor in getting sound sleep. B_3 also tends to help with blood sugar balance, which can help with sleep (and control hunger).

Vitamin B_6 is required for the production of serotonin, that "calming hormone" that helps control mood, appetite, sleep patterns, and even sensitivity to pain.

Vitamin B_{12} appears to help some people regain normal sleep patterns after bouts with insomnia and frequent awakening during the night.

Folic Acid deficiency can cause insomnia, so having a sufficient supply is key. Remember to review anything you are thinking about taking with your doctor to make sure you are not taking too much, that it will not interact with what you are taking (medications) or will not do damage to current medical conditions.

For some, the B vitamins can be stimulating, so either try taking them a few hours before bed to see how you respond, or take your vitamins earlier in the day. Foods richest in B vitamins include whole grains, cereal, nuts, broccoli, and potatoes.

Calcium: Calcium is a natural relaxant with a calming effect on the nervous system; in fact, calcium is one of the most important minerals for proper functioning of the nervous system. Calcium can also help regulate the heart and blood pressure. Unfortunately, many people don't get enough calcium in their diet (especially if they avoid dairy), or they can have problems digesting and absorbing it well. Drinking carbonated beverages, for example, can strip away the calcium your body wants to retain for building bones and preventing osteoporosis.

Calcium can be taken in 500-milligram doses or less between meals, and should be taken in conjunction with magnesium and potassium to help your system absorb it.

Magnesium: Several studies have shown that magnesium can assist your sleep, whether you're a chronic insomniac or experience poor sleep on occasion. It should be taken in balanced proportions of two parts calcium and one part magnesium.

Zinc: Zinc deficiencies have been linked to insomnia, among many medical problems, in several studies. Make sure you are getting your daily allotment of zinc.

Copper and Iron: When you're deprived of normal amounts of copper or iron, sleep can be seriously affected. Iron is known to be one of the many things that can cause restless legs syndrome. In fact, I have had several patients whose "weird feeling" in their legs simply vanishes after beginning iron supplementation.

The bottom line: Invest in a good multivitamin with at least all of these vitamins and minerals present. If you feel you need to supplement with more than just the daily allowance suggested by the government ("Recommended Daily Allowances"), discuss this with your doctor. Some supplements, like copper and iron, should only be taken under the supervision of a physician.

Indigestion and acid reflux got your sleep? If you're a victim of GERD (gastroesophageal reflux disease) or just experience it on occasion because of what you've eaten, there's more you can do than just avoid certain foods at dinner and be sure to eat well in advance of bedtime. As previously mentioned, a lot of digestion is based on—and dependent upon—gravity. So when you are lying down, the contents of your stomach can push against the valve between the esophagus and stomach and end up going the wrong direction, giving you that painful "heartburn." The box on page 117 contains tips for combating the effects of GERD that are very effective and quite simple, and the two most useful tricks are the following:

- Avoid lying down for two to three hours after eating.
- Raise the head of your bed six to eight inches by placing blocks underneath the bed frame or by using a foam wedge under the head of your mattress.

Action Reminder

Today's relaxation technique: Drink a cup of hot herbal, non-caffeinated tea about an hour before bedtime. Do not forget to do at least one stretching exercise and a deep breathing exercise. Perform your Sun Salutes in the morning.

What to record in your diary at the start of Day 7:
- lights-out time
- how long you think it took you to fall asleep
- the time you woke up
- the quality of your sleep (rate 1–10)
- how refreshed you feel in the a.m. (rate 1–10)
- On a scale of 1–10, how relaxed did your bedtime technique make you feel? Which stretches and/or guided imagery ideas did you try?
- How much:
  ➤ caffeine you ingested and when
  ➤ nicotine you ingested and when
  ➤ alcohol you ingested and when
- What's left to do to your room to make it a better sleep environment?
- Did you remember to do some stretching, such as the Sun Salute, in the morning?

- What was the time of your last meal? Was it at least four hours before bed?
- What did you eat?
- Have you gone out and bought a good multivitamin?

NIGHT 7: FIND THE RIGHT TIME TO EXERCISE

Myth Buster: *Exercise at the end of the day is always a bad idea for getting to sleep.* This is not necessarily true. For many, exercise provides the perfect preamble for sound sleep.

Exercise and Temperature: The Warm-up Cooldown Solution

As you would expect, aerobic exercise increases your body temperature, which then subsequently cools down over several hours, dropping to a nadir that you could not have reached without that physical activity. This cooldown also happens right before you fall asleep. Your core body temperature begins to fall, which signals to your brain that it's time to go to bed. Of course, exercise is not the only way to get your body warmed up—you can simply take a hot bath. But exercise can also affect your circadian rhythm, as we've already discussed in Chapter 6. We know, for example, that aerobic exercise helps increase Stages III and IV (deep) sleep in some people. The issue, then, becomes timing the exercise right during the day in preparation to sleep.

Getting regular exercise as part of a healthy lifestyle is, for many, "easier said than done." In other words, fewer and fewer people are scheduling physical activity into their busy—often sedentary—days, and if they do attempt an exercise routine, it's for weight-loss purposes only. We've already covered how exercise and sleep work together in Chapter 6. It can't be said enough: Exercise has few downsides, and almost no downsides for sleep purposes so long as it's timed correctly. An intense workout scheduled perfectly will ready your body for sleep, ease your tensions and stress, and usher in quality deep sleep. Now it's time to get you moving and experimenting with timing your exercise properly. From Day 7 onward through the rest of the month, you're going to determine: 1) what hour during the day is optimal for you to be exercising; 2) what level of intensity you should practice; and 3) whether exercise has a positive or negative impact on your sleep. Not everyone will have the same answers. If you are the type of person who gets energized or becomes more alert after exercise, it may be wise not to exercise in the evening. Regular exercise in the morning, on the other hand, can help with sleep problems.

PRACTICAL QUIZ

Where do you fall? Circle the statements that best describe you. If you circle more than two under "p.m. exerciser," experiment with afternoon/evening exercise first. If you circle more than three under "a.m. exerciser," then try a morning workout.

a.m. exerciser	p.m. exerciser (3 hours before bed)
After exercise, I feel energized.	After exercise, I feel relaxed and sleepy.
I have a nervous habit of tapping my foot.	
I wake up with a brain full of thoughts.	I cannot turn off my mind.
I have a hard time focusing during the day.	
I am a generally happy person.	I have more down or blue time than normal.
I have many activities.	I do not participate in activities much.
I am an early A.M. person.	I am a night owl.

If you don't consider yourself a physically active person and hardly ever participate in an exercise routine, that's okay. Just try to pick some of these statements and see where you fall.

If you're a seasoned exerciser or athlete, you may not need to do much work in this department, especially if your exercise habits work for you and coordinate with your sleep habits. You may, however, wish to use this month to play around with *when* you perform your exercise to see if you can time it better for supporting sound sleep. For example, if you're a lark who loves the morning hours but who puts off the exercise hour until after work, try scheduling your workout in the morning instead of later on. You might discover that it's easier to wind down in the evening and easily fall asleep at night in preparation for the early morning. Also, if you are getting up at the crack of dawn to exercise and are missing out on extra sleep, that's not healthy, either. You may find it beneficial to shift your physical fitness routine to the afternoon or early evening. In some cases you can break up your exercise and do only certain exercises in the afternoon and others in the morning. This will allow you to get your workout and still maintain optimal sleep time. (Remember: The benefits from exercise are cumulative, so you don't necessarily have to complete a full one-hour workout in the same chunk of time. You can space it out throughout your day.)

For those who've never implemented a regular exercise routine, start by scheduling in twenty-minute walks at least three times a week. Go easy on yourself if you're not physically fit and be patient with the process of getting into shape. It's wise to discuss your goals with your doctor first, especially if you have back, leg, lung, heart, or any medical issues that would make exercise dangerous. Aim to establish a regular exercise program that increases your heart rate and gets your body moving, reaching, stretching, and feeling great. Even if you just take the stairs or park your car at the edge of the lot, you have to start somewhere, and remember you are going to get better sleep because of this.

Taking your pulse. Learn how to take your pulse so you can test yourself at the beginning and end of a walk or other exercise. Trace a line with your index and second finger from the corner of your eye down to your jawline, then go just beneath it to your neck. Gently press until you feel a pulsation. Now look at your watch and count the pulses for six seconds. Multiply this number by ten and you have your pulse. Record your pulse in your diary. Your pulse after exercise should be between twenty and forty beats higher than your resting pulse, the pulse you recorded prior to exercise. If you're not getting your pulse up, increase the intensity of your workout. If it's greater than forty to fifty beats higher, consult your doctor and decrease the intensity of your workout.

THE IMPACT OF SUNLIGHT

Let's also not forget that sunlight during exercise can help entrain your circadian rhythm. As I've already pointed out, it's imperative that you get your daily dose of sunlight. Combining sunlight and a small amount of exercise every morning can work wonders on your body's rhythms—not to mention elevate your mood. Here are a few ideas:

1. If you have a dog that needs walking, make a point of being the dog walker at least a few times a week in the morning. Time your walks so you get some sun (this can be difficult during winter months when the sun rises late) with your walking.

2. Start a morning walking program where you take fifteen to twenty minutes to walk around your neighborhood and soak in that morning sunlight. Pick up the newspaper on your way back into the house. Or, if your mail arrives in the morning, mix a small walk with clearing out your mailbox when you get back.

Action Reminder

Today's relaxation technique: Download my free program that walks you through a muscle relaxation exercise on my site: www.soundsleep solutions.com. This program should be listened to in the dim light with headphones on if needed. Since this is a day where you begin your exercise program, it will be essential that you stretch. Also include some deep-breathing exercises with guided imagery, if necessary. Do your Sun Salutes again in the morning.

What to record in your diary at the start of Day 8:
- lights-out time
- how long you think it took you to fall asleep
- the time you woke up
- the quality of your sleep (rate 1–10)
- how refreshed you feel in the a.m. (rate 1–10)
- On a scale of 1–10, how relaxed did your bedtime technique make you feel? Which stretches and/or guided imagery ideas did you try?

- How much:
  - ➤ caffeine you ingested and when
  - ➤ nicotine you ingested and when
  - ➤ alcohol you ingested and when
- What's left to do to your room to make it a better sleep environment?
- Did you remember to do some stretching, such as the Sun Salute, in the morning?
- What was the time of your last meal? Was it at least four hours before bed?
- What did you eat?
- Did you exercise yesterday? If so, what did you do and when did you do it?

Congratulations. You've just completed the first week of your sleep boot camp.

SoundSleepSolutions.com

Don't forget to check out my Web site at www.soundsleepsolutions.com. There, you can write to me about your personal experiences with sleep, share your own tips on an active message board, and ask questions. I'll post the most frequently asked questions with their answers and possible solutions. Your questions will contribute to an online and active Troubleshooting Guide.

CHAPTER 9

Week 2: Review, Rework, and Revive

Last week I exposed you to a variety of new lifestyle ideas to try that should help rescue your sleep. But as you can guess, it takes more than just one week to see results, and you have to continue to experiment and be your own sleep therapist in the coming weeks.

If you haven't managed to get through the first week as successfully as you'd like, or if you missed a day of the program and are "off-schedule," that's okay. An alternative to doing this 28-night program day after day (with new elements to add each day) is to take each main focus and use an entire week to devote to that focus. For example, you can take the whole first week to concentrate solely on your sleep cycles and figure out what's the best time for you to go to bed and wake up. Then, use the whole second week to focus mainly on establishing a bedtime routine while you continue to pay attention to your sleep-wake cycles. Defining your personal sleep profile—the hour that you should go to bed based on sleep cycles and morning wake-up calls—can be a difficult homework assignment, especially if you're extremely out of sync with your body clock. You might not want to think about anything else until you've gotten your sleep-wake cycle understood. So feel free to use the program's time line as a rough sketch only, and proceed when you feel ready to learn more and progress to more advanced lifestyle modifications. Obviously, this time line will last longer than twenty-eight nights.

In this chapter I'll assume you've gotten through your first week and have gathered enough information and recorded it in your sleep diary to make some solid evaluations.

Emerging from Boot Camp

Myth Buster: *People sleep better in the warmer temperatures than in the cooler temperatures.* Actually, the reverse is true: People sleep better in cooler temps. So, while you might prefer your day to be a balmy eighty degrees, at night your body would much prefer the cooler side of sixty-five to seventy-two degrees Fahrenheit. Being warm under the covers in a chilly bedroom has its benefits.

NIGHT 8: A STUDY OF WEEK 1 AT A GLANCE

It's time to go back to the sleep diary you've been keeping for the last week and plug some information into this chart.

Remember what you should have put in your sleep diary:

- lights-out time
- how long you think it took you to fall asleep
- the time you woke up
- the quality of your sleep (rate 1–10)
- how refreshed you feel in the A.M. (rate 1–10)

	Day 1	Day 2	Day 3	Day 4	Day 5	Day 6	Day 7
Lights-out							
Time to Sleep							
Wake Time							
Sleep Quality							
Refreshed							

First, examine your bedtime. Were you able to complete any of the experiments that first day? If yes and you arrived at a proper bedtime, how many nights were you able to follow that time schedule? If it was more than four, you are doing great. If you could only adhere to your bedtime three nights this past week, that's good, but set your goal for this next week at between four and five nights. If you only managed to get to bed twice this past week at the right time, then you need to look at what priority you are placing on sleep. Is it really that important to you? If it is, then you really need to start that bedtime routine and get yourself to bed on time. If sleep is a priority but the bedtime feels off, try another one of the experiments. For example, if you have discovered that you are an owl, push your bedtime about half an hour later and your wake time fifteen minutes later. See if that helps. Enlist everyone in the house—tell them you will stop being grumpy and moody if they will just help you with this program.

Next, on average, how long is it taking to fall asleep? If it's longer than thirty minutes, your bedtime is still too early or your body has not had the time to adjust to its new circadian or biological rhythm. More than thirty minutes to fall asleep means you need to make your bedtime fifteen minutes later.

Are you able to wake at the same time every morning, including the weekends? If not, remember: **Your wake time is one of the most important factors in this program.** If you can do nothing else, make sure you are waking at the same time.

Has the rating of your quality of sleep improved over the week? (Are your numbers getting higher?) Have you felt more refreshed over the week? (Are your numbers getting higher?) If they have not, **Do not worry.** Many of my patients have said it gets worse before it gets better. Do not be discouraged. If your numbers remain the same, give it more time.

Jane's Story

Jane R. came to me in the clinic a mess. Constantly exhausted, she told me that she felt like her life was out of control and that there was little she could do about it. She was convinced that if she could get enough sleep she would feel better, and possibly good enough to get some of her other responsibilities done. Jane had left her job to raise her kids at home while her husband worked twice as hard to make the family's ends meet. I asked Jane to start a sleep diary because when I first saw her, she wasn't even able to recall the times when she had gone to sleep the previous two days. What we discovered over time was that she was going to bed between 10 P.M. and 2 A.M.; her wake-up time depended upon her kids' school commitments and her husband's morning schedule. Sometimes he could go in late to work so she could sleep.

Jane's irregular sleep schedule was taking its toll. Together we decided to come up with constant bedtimes and wake times for her to stick to. She was so tired that she was willing to try anything. Jane discussed these ideas with her husband, friends, and kids to make sure everyone was on board for supporting her schedule. It had to be a team effort. We chose 10:30 P.M. as the time for her to get ready for bed, then be in bed by 11:00 to be asleep by 11:30. Assuming she could fall asleep by 11:30, we chose 6:30 A.M. as her wake-up time.

The first week was unsuccessful and, in a word, disastrous. Because organization clearly wasn't her forte and her husband was out of town, she only got to bed on time twice. She got to bed very late in the first half of the week, and then only got to bed by 11 toward the end of the week—solely as a result of sheer exhaustion. But the turnaround came as soon as she recognized, through her journaling, that when she got to bed on time, she got up naturally within fifteen minutes of her wake-up time and felt more relaxed and refreshed on those days than on any other day of the week. This validated how important it was for her to respect her bedtime. She then worked very hard at practicing her bedtime routine and making it a priority in the family. After about six weeks, Jane reported feeling like a new person. She said she owed a lot to her family, who kept her on track and helped her avoid falling back into her old routine of staying up late to finish house chores. Today when Jane feels the urge to stay up past her bedtime, she reminds herself of what it was like to be worn out and on the edge of "losing it" all day. That single memory alone makes the decision to call it a day and hit the hay easy.

Next, how many hours as a whole do you think you got? Compared with national standards, parents get an average of six hours and forty minutes of sleep a night, plus or minus twenty minutes. A person who docks only five hours of sleep each night must recognize he or she is far below the norm and may need to make greater changes if five hours doesn't feel like enough.

Evaluate your bedtime and wake time:

Does this bed time feel correct to you?	Yes/No
Does it need to be earlier?	Yes/No
Does it need to be later?	Yes/No
Is this because you need more time at night for chores?	Yes/No

Did you notice a trend that your ratings increased on the days after you were able to keep your new bedtime? If yes, then you appear to have found what you need; if no, try one of the other experiments from Day 1. If all of them say the same time, that's okay. Your body is simply adjusting to this new time and it may take a week or so longer.

Continue your diary and remember that *wake time* is the most important variable. That might seem strange since we are talking about bedtimes right now, so let me explain: Your wake time is when your body resets itself every day. So this must be the most consistent starting point for everyone. With this consistency we can then work backward to bedtime. We will revisit these timing issues again on the fifteenth day.

CHECKING IN ON YOUR PARTNER

Recall Chapter 3 where we covered tricks for dealing with a bed partner who disrupts your sleep. Does your bed partner understand how his or her sleep habits affect you? Have you evaluated new ways to make you and your bed partner sleep-compatible? Which problems are the most apparent—snoring, restlessness, a different sleep schedule? Review the ideas shared in Chapter 3's Action Plan and implement those ideas now, if you haven't already done so. Focus on the ways in which you can set your bedroom up for accommodating two different types of sleepers.

Keep pets off the bed. Does your pet sleep with you? This, too, may cause you to awaken during the night, either from allergies or pet movements. Fido and Fluffy might be better off on the floor or in their own bed than on your sheets.

> **Stagger bedtimes.** If your bed partner prevents you from getting to sleep, try going to sleep first, then have your partner join you after you have fallen into a deep sleep.

Checklist of 10 Things to Be Aware of During This Week

- ❑ Bedtime routine
  - ➤ One-hour downtime
  - ➤ Relaxation/meditation techniques
  - ➤ Deep breathing
- ❑ Get to bed on time! Wake up on time!
- ❑ Ensure you get an ample supply of vitamins and minerals.
- ❑ Watch caffeine intake in the afternoon.
- ❑ Beware of nicotine and alcohol.
- ❑ Curb consumptions of foods likely to cause indigestion or acid reflux.
- ❑ Get exposure to morning sunlight.
- ❑ Experiment with time of exercise.
- ❑ Create the ideal sleep environment.
- ❑ Do your Sun Salutes in the mornings.

Nights 9–14

These days mimic each of Nights 2 through 7; you'll review what you've tried and how well you've been able to keep up with the new or modified routine over the past eight days. As you evaluate yourself in the coming days, take note of the boxes called **Up the Ante** and see if you can take your new sleep-friendly habits even further.

NIGHT 9: REVIEW BEDTIME ROUTINE

> **Myth Buster:** *It takes a long time to reset the body's internal clock.* In actuality, the body resets its own internal clock each day with the help of sunlight. If you cannot access sunlight, any light—especially one that mimics the intensity of sunlight—will do. Exercise can also help reset the body's clock.

Ask yourself the following questions:

- Have you set aside at least one hour before your bedtime?
- During the last week did you do any of the following activities within an hour before bed?
  - ➤ writing/receiving e-mail, surfing the Web, or playing computer games
  - ➤ paying bills
  - ➤ watching TV
  - ➤ having important conversations with your spouse
  - ➤ eating or drinking (except water)
  - ➤ reading or referring to anything work related, such as newspaper articles, manuals, textbooks, PowerPoint presentations, and so on
- If you answered yes to any of the above, your goal for the next week is to find a better time to do these activities outside of that sacred one hour before bedtime.

The TV Question: If you are one of those people who simply cannot turn his or her mind off without help from watching TV, or if you have always slept with the TV on and it's conditioned you to fall asleep more easily, then you may need to have the TV on as a method of relaxation. Several of my patients claim that to disallow TV prior to bedtime would wreak more havoc on their ability to fall asleep. If that describes you, then okay. You can continue to watch TV, but you must have a TV timer set. The changes in programming and advertisements that occur through the night with varying volumes can disturb your sleep.

- During the first half of your Power-Down Hour, did you finish any mindless chores you needed to do?
  - ➤ Did these chores take more than thirty minutes?
  - ➤ If so, were you still able to get into bed on time? If not, then you need to either delegate the chores to someone else or start earlier.
- Were you able to complete your hygiene activities: brushing your teeth, washing your face, taking nighttime medications, slipping into your loose-fitting bedclothes, and turning off all the lights in your bedroom, closets, and bathrooms except for the night-lights?
  - ➤ Did this take more than fifteen minutes? If so, trim your list or start ten minutes earlier.

Evaluate your bedtime routine:

1. Do you like having a routine?   Yes/No
2. Does it help you get in the right frame of mind to sleep?   Yes/No
3. Do other people in your house respect your routine?   Yes/No

If the routine is helping you, you are on your way to setting the stage for a better night's sleep. If you feel the routine is creating more stress, review it again and try to see why. This section is critical for your success. Sure, there will be times when you cannot follow your routine for whatever reason, but you must have some wind-down time before bed, to signal your body to get ready for sleep.

Reminders:

- Do not forget to do your deep-breathing exercises and your Sun Salutes in the morning.
- Did you get your dose of sunlight today?
- Did you take your multivitamin today?

John's Story

John M. came to me with some mild sleep issues. He didn't meet criteria for a formal sleep disorder, but he frequently had problems getting enough sleep. Sometimes he worried about work and his job; other times he stayed up late watching football or a favorite movie. When John and I spoke about his sleep deprivation, he said he didn't feel as though it was "all that bad." I probed him further and got to the root of the problem: He admitted to having marital troubles that drove him to avoid going to bed while his wife was awake. So he was putting off his bedtime until later in the night. He also mentioned that he didn't feel like he was connecting with his wife anymore.

I suggested that we bring in his wife to tackle his sleep issues as a team. I knew that if we enlisted her help and got her involved, they would be approaching the problem in a way that could bring them closer together—and get him into bed earlier. As it turned out, his wife was very agreeable. I helped them create a list of chores, and we cited which ones could be done together. John's wife was happy to see that he was willing to help out, and John enjoyed spending that time with his wife. Now they end up in bed at the same time, and report that the spark has returned to their marriage.

Up the Ante: Take your most time-consuming task you do each night and make it someone else's responsibility. For example, if you're always the one to clean up the kitchen or take the trash out, and those chores frequently cut into your Power-Down Hour, enlist the help of a teenager or a spouse.

NIGHT 10: REVIEW CAFFEINE, ALCOHOL, AND NICOTINE

Myth Buster: *Because melatonin is sold without a prescription, it's totally safe.* To many people's surprise, melatonin is not regulated by the FDA yet can be readily found over-the-counter in drug and health food stores. Taking supplemental melatonin, which is a hormone that regulates sleep-wake cycles, can be dangerous. In Europe, for instance, melatonin is sold by prescription only. (See Chapter 11 for more information.)

All that you consume during the day, from medications and supplements to food and beverages, can have a direct impact on your sleep. The three biggest issues, as we've seen, are caffeine, alcohol, and nicotine. Refer to your diary and ask yourself these questions:

- Alcohol: Were you able to follow the guidelines?
  - ➤ How much did you consume over the course of the week? If you did not drink each evening, on the nights that you did, how did you sleep?
  - ➤ At what time did you stop drinking compared to your bedtime? Remember: For every drink, you will need to leave about an hour for it to be metabolized.
  - ➤ Did you wake up in the middle of the night or have restless sleep after drinking?
- Nicotine
  - ➤ Did you try to quit or curb your smoking? If yes and it worked, that's good news. If yes and it didn't work, remember that I gave you permission to continue smoking so withdrawal effects wouldn't counter your efforts to improve your sleep habits.

➤ Could you avoid having that last cigarette close to bedtime?
- Caffeine:
    - ➤ Were you able to identify your caffeine cutoff point as described on page 187?
    - ➤ Were you also able to step down your caffeine consumption so that as you progressed throughout the day, the caffeine content of your beverages decreased?

Relaxation Check:

On the third day, your relaxation exercise was to write down your biggest stressors of the day and see if you could come up with a solution to each of them. Was that exercise helpful? If so, consider taking that exercise to new heights (see Up the Ante) and develop a worry journal.

Up the Ante: Start a Worry Journal

Go buy a small journal for yourself that you call My Worry Journal. Use it for one thing only: listing out your thoughts and worries, especially the ones that bombard you at night as you try to wind down and fall asleep. Include one possible solution to each worry, even if that means writing "take care of tomorrow." Keep the worry journal beside your bed. They now make pens that light up, so you don't have to turn on a light to write your worries down. If you spring to wakefulness in the middle of the night with a terrible, stressful thought, you can write that down in your journal, too. Then put the journal away and practice a few relaxation techniques.

Reminders:
- Do not forget to do your deep-breathing exercises and your Sun Salutes in the morning.
- Did you get your dose of sunlight today?
- Did you take your multivitamin today?

NIGHT 11: REVIEW BEDROOM ENVIRONMENT

Myth Buster: *Polarfleece or silk sheets are always a bad idea because they can retain too much heat and make you uncomfortable.* Temperature is a very subjective topic when it comes to sleeping conditions. While most find light cotton the best fabric for bedding and, in particular, sheets, some do love their heavier fleece and silks during the winter months.

Recall that on the third day I asked you to read something light and fun or really boring prior to going to bed. Were you able to identify good reading material? Were you able to complete the task? On a scale of 1 to 10, how relaxed were you after spending time reading? (Remember: You should be keeping this info in your diary.) Did you notice the quality of your sleep change?

If you felt this exercise was helpful, try taking it to new heights.

Up the Ante: Bedtime Reading

The best bedtime reading often entails the following:

- trade journals and textbooks, as long as you are not that interested in the subject
- books with short chapters, or magazines with short articles
- anything truly technical in nature

  Make sure you use a book light and not an overhead light.

Quiz to assess your bedroom environment:

1. Have you changed the bulb wattage or installed dimmer switches? If so, score +1.

2. Is your furniture arranged so that your bed is away from direct sunlight or nearby noise? If so, score +1.

3. Are your wall hangings and adornments calm and peaceful? If yes, score +1.

4. Did you at least turn or flip (remember: not if it's a pillow top) your mattress? If yes, score +1.

5. Are your bedding linens clean, soft, and comfortable? If yes, score +1.

6. Are your pillows, blankets, and covers allergen-free? Comfortable? And have you done the dead-pillow test and gotten rid of the dead pillows? Whichever you've answered yes to, score +1 (total points available is +3 here).

7. Have you gotten the computer monitors out of the room? (Only if they were in there before do you get a +1.)

8. Have you taken steps to decrease the source and intensity of sound (natural and artificial, including TV)? If yes, score +1.

9. Are the odors pleasant? If yes, score +1.

10. Is the air quality good? If yes, score +1.

11. Is the temperature between sixty-five and seventy degrees Fahrenheit, with a humidity of about 65 percent? If yes, score +1.

12. Have you cleared the clutter from your bedroom? If yes, score +1.

If your score is 9–14, then you have truly begun to create a sleep sanctuary. Great work. Keep going.

If your score is 5–8, then you have made some good progress. If you feel like you've done enough and you're satisfied, you can stop. But you are on the verge of an ever greater sleep-friendly bedroom.

If your score is 4 or lower, my first question is: Why? Most of these steps should not take too much financial resources to perform. You need to tell yourself that sound sleep cannot come without a sound sleep environment.

Reminders:
- Do not forget to do your deep-breathing exercises and your Sun Salutes in the morning.
- Did you get your dose of sunlight today?
- Did you take your multivitamin today?

Jill's Story

Jill J. complained that she didn't sleep well, and was tired of getting so-so sleep. She was a bit high-strung, but on the whole a happy person who enjoyed cooking and decorating her home. I could tell she was the type who liked to keep her home orderly, clean, and supremely thought-out, design-wise. Her job made it difficult to get all the household chores done, which made her feel unsettled when she climbed into bed. Even though she had removed all of the clutter from the bedroom, and changed the pictures on the walls so they all were serene and peaceful, she realized once we got talking that she had a long way to go on perfecting her sleep environment.

After sitting down and sketching out her room, we discovered several different areas that needed attention. First we created a shopping list of items she needed to purchase, which we then prioritized based on 1) price and 2) the likelihood of it helping her and her husband's sleep. Next we decided how fancy she wanted to make her bedroom, tossing around options from Wal-Mart to Neiman Marcus—all of which would be helpful and miraculously fit into her budget. Finally, we put together a time line and wrote down any obstacles that could prevent her from getting, hanging, or fixing what we'd agreed upon. Then Jill was off and on her way.

Today she resides in a perfect sleep sanctuary. She and her husband have never slept better.

NIGHT 12: REVIEW BEDTIME AND WAKING STRETCHING

Myth Buster: *Any physical activity, even light stretching, can inhibit sleep.* Not so! One of the best ways to relax and prepare your mind and body for sleep is to do a few yoga-like poses either on the floor next to your bed or even on it.

Given the stretches and relaxation techniques described starting on the fifth day, which ones did you find helpful? Did you find at least two that worked well for you? Were there any that you liked or did not like? (Recap of techniques: Relaxed Standing Forward Bend; the Point-to-Point Release; the Cobbler's Pose with Head Rolls; Deep Breathing; the Cat Stretch; the Sponge; and the Relaxation Pose.)

Once you have identified two stretches you enjoy and which help you lose your mind to sleep, add them to your routine every night.

If doing the Sun Salutes in the morning isn't your thing and you'd rather do something else upon awakening in the morning, try scheduling in your "sun time" here by stepping outside for a ten-to-fifteen-minute walk at a brisk pace. After your walk, do some stretching to loosen up your legs and arms. Remember to practice deep belly breathing.

Up the Ante: Stretching for Two!

If you and your bed partner share similar bedtimes, you might try stretching together or giving each other massages. Your partner can add weight or more resistance to your stretching exercises, which can help you relax deeper. Bear in mind, however, that massages can be preludes to more intimate moments. If this is a time within your hour before bed and sexual activity can rev you up, remember there are more relaxing forms of sexual activity you and your partner can engage in.

Reminders:
- Did you take your multivitamin today?

NIGHT 13: REVIEW DIET CHOICES

Myth Buster: *A large lunch will induce a "food coma," putting you to sleep soon thereafter.* The afternoon lull typically hits after we've eaten lunch. But that lull isn't created by what we've eaten; rather, it correlates to a biological rhythm whereby our core body temperature drops in the mid-afternoon, causing us to feel sleepy.

Changing your diet can be a difficult challenge that requires effort and attention day in and day out—especially if your eating habits are well-ingrained. Ask yourself:

- Have you been able to focus on my food guidelines?
- Have you changed the time of your dinner?
- Have you changed the amount of your dinner?
- Have you changed the content of your dinner?
- If you suffer from acid reflux or GERD, did your condition subside at all?
- Are you in need of a bedtime snack?
  - ➤ If so, are you making smart choices and going for calcium- and protein-rich snacks with a little carbohydrates?
- Did you find that drinking a cup of hot herbal, non-caffeinated tea was helpful?

Reminders:
- Incorporate two stretches into your bedtime routine.
- Do not forget to do your deep-breathing exercises and your Sun Salutes or a walk in the morning.
- Did you get your dose of sunlight today?
- Did you take your multivitamin today?

NIGHT 14: REVIEW EXERCISE ROUTINE

Myth Buster: *Vigorous exercise before bed is the worst thing that an overly anxious person can do.* Although it was originally thought that exercise before bed could negatively impact sleep, some research shows that in anxious individuals, exercise before bed can be quite calming.

I performed an experiment as a graduate student when reviewing the effects of exercise on highly anxious individuals. My fellow researchers and I found that exercise relieves anxiety more in highly anxious individuals than in normal individuals. So naturally the next question would seem to be: Does the decline in anxiety translate to better sleep just before bed? To date I am unaware of a formal experiment that can answer this question, but I do have Sarah's story to share with anecdotal evidence.

Sarah was a self-admitted stress mess. She explained to me in a session that throughout her life she had always been someone with a high anxiety level. She could get utterly stressed out about many things, but the biggest instigator for her was stress related to being late. Her tardiness appeared to increase her stress, and even if she could meet her deadlines, once she was stressed, she had a hard time letting it go. She also told me that by the end of the day her stress level was so high, it prevented her from falling asleep. It wasn't uncommon for her to make lists of the things she needed to do and then proceed to stay up late trying to relax. She found herself in cycles of staying up too late, then sleeping in too late, which shifted her schedule off for the day . . . thus recycling the stress all over again.

Sarah and I worked on several solutions. First we focused on time management and organization. Sarah had to learn how to give herself permission to wind down in the hours before bedtime and turn her brain off once she got into bed. Next we worked on her wake-up time because this appeared to be a significant stressor for her. I asked her to go out and buy pillow speakers for her alarm, since she often slept through her usual alarm. Once Sarah was on a regular schedule, things began to fall into place for her, but she still experienced a significant amount of low-level underlying stress.

At that point we explored stress relief programs and decided upon exercise as a good place to start. Sarah began walking in the mornings to get sunlight and accomplished two tasks by making a few telephone calls while exercising. Thus if she was running late she could contact people and reduce her stress. On days when it was impossible to schedule in an a.m. walk, we decided that part of her power-down hour could be devoted to exercise. I explained to her the benefits of aerobic exercise (more so than what she was getting through leisure walks), and she shared that she'd been thinking about restarting an exercise routine again, anyhow (she'd been a regular exerciser previously, but hadn't participated in a regular routine in a very long time, so she felt like she was starting over). She worried that the exercise would be too stimulating, but after testing it out a few nights a week, she reported getting a better night's sleep on the evenings when she exercised and feeling more refreshed those next mornings.

Nailing down the best time of day for you to exercise may take time and further experimentation. If this is the first time you've embarked on an exercise program (or you simply haven't exercised regularly in a long time), you may find that timing the exercise right isn't as big of a deal as just finding any time to schedule a workout into your day. That's okay. Be patient with yourself and go at your own pace. You can always focus on timing your workouts better a bit later on. Your first goal should be starting a regular exercise routine, and your second goal should be timing it right.

At this juncture, ask yourself:

- Did you start an exercise program once you had gotten the thumbs-up from your doctor?
- Are you participating in it at least three times a week?

- Does your workout routine involve cardio (to get your heart rate up), resistance training (use of free weights), and some stretching for flexibility?
- Do you notice a change in your sleep habits based on your physical activity alone?
- Do you notice a change in your sleep habits based on *when* you exercise?

Remember: An exercise routine needn't be overly strenuous and ambitious. A brisk thirty-minute walk will suffice, plus some use of weights and stretching. If you need the motivation of others around you, try a group class such as body sculpting, step aerobics, indoor cycling, or form your own group of weekday walkers and weekend hikers. You don't need to join a gym, buy a piece of equipment, or visit a fancy studio to get a high-quality workout, as there are lots of options—from DVDs you can use in the comfort of your home, to even virtual workouts you can do while online with others. The only item you may need to invest in is a good pair of sneakers or running shoes.

Let's quickly evaluate your relaxation techniques again:

- Did you download my program that walks you through a muscle relaxation exercise for free on my site: www.soundsleep solutions.com?
- Did it relax you and make you feel better?
- Were you able to fall asleep and stay asleep?
- How relaxed were you in the morning?

Reminders:
- Incorporate two stretches into your bedtime routine.
- Do not forget to do your deep-breathing exercises and your Sun Salutes or go for a walk in the morning.
- Did you get your dose of sunlight today?
- Did you take your multivitamin today?

Bravo! You've completed Week 2. As you think back to the past seven days, ask yourself two questions:

1. What was the most difficult part of the program this past week?
2. What was the most rewarding part of the program this past week?

Take your answers and be mindful of them as you begin your third week. If, at any time, you feel that this program is moving too fast for you, make your next steps a little slower and consider following the alternate program described at the start of this chapter. Or, take whatever you found to be the most difficult challenge this past week and use the entire upcoming week to focus on just that task. Keep in mind that the modifications you're making day after day are cumulative. If concentrating on just two or three lifestyle modifications is your limit at this point, such as curbing your thirst for caffeine and getting to bed on time, that's okay. I want you to go at your own pace. Listen to your body and follow its lead. You know that crash diets don't work, and neither does making radical lifestyle changes even if they are in the best interests of your sleep. The more you give your body time to adjust to newly established habits, the greater likelihood that you'll continue to practice good sleep habits, be able to maintain healthy sleep hygiene . . . and the better you'll look and feel year after year, night after night . . . day after day.

CHAPTER 10

Weeks 3 and 4:
Setting It All in Motion

When Katherine first came to me, she was in trouble. Faced with a very demanding job as an ER nurse and as a mom with two kids at home (ages eight and fourteen), Katherine was referred to me by her doctor, who believed Katherine's debilitating, chronic migraines were linked to inadequate sleep. Ever since going back to work after the birth of her second child, she'd experienced long bouts of insomnia and had a terrible time getting up in the morning. Katherine never felt rested and, combined with the stress of the day, she was always on the verge of a monstrous migraine. Although she had suffered from migraines since she was a teenager, now Katherine was experiencing them about twice a week; they ran her life, often leaving her unable to work and be available for her family. She had to take beta-blockers to help prevent the headaches, which always made her sleepy, and then very strong vasoconstrictors to ease the migraines, which always stimulated her. These medicines were not a long-term solution. Katherine was determined to put an end to the cycle of worrying about a migraine attack and then treating one. She wanted our clinic to put her on a regimen of prescription sleeping pills, with the idea that once she got adequate sleep, the migraines would disappear. I disagreed, at least in part.

My first course of action was to evaluate Katherine's daily routines. Although she was up by 5:30 A.M., she admitted to being more of an owl than a lark. When I asked her to pinpoint when the migraines seemed to happen more frequently, she replied, "When I came back after maternity leave. I took on double shifts and found myself in the ER in the middle of the night—which I'd never done before. My body always felt out of whack."

Migraine headaches can be worsened by sleep deprivation, so we knew we had to fix her constant sleep debt. It was also important to balance her sleep schedule because, in some cases, too much sleep can agitate the problem, too. With Katherine, we relied on the experiments in Day 1 to locate a good bedtime and wake time for her. It took us about a week and a half, experimenting with her going to bed a bit later and sleeping a bit longer. Eventually we found her "zone." Once that had been established, we turned to another popular external factor that was making her headaches worse: alcohol. We spoke for a long time about this subject. Katherine had always enjoyed a nice glass of wine with dinner and found it was one of the few pleasures that relaxed her. But we didn't need to ax the wine entirely from her menu. What we did instead was experiment with various types of wine and, not to my surprise, we found that those with fewer tannins were less likely to give her a "beginner's headache," as she called it. And she almost never got a headache from wine if she was following her sleep schedule. We also spoke at length with a prescribing doctor to make sure she could have wine while taking this medication.

Next we focused on her bedroom and discussed what factors were preventing her from getting to sleep at the right time. One was noise from her teenage daughter talking on the phone in the adjacent room into the wee hours of the night. Katherine then tried several noise machines, but settled on a pair of noise-rated earplugs. This way, she knew her daughter was fine but did not have to listen to her all night.

The discovery process with Katherine took time and patience, but we eventually determined all of the issues crippling her sleep and we addressed them one by one. She experienced several migraine headaches along the way, and we occasionally had to stall treatment in order for her to get through them. At one point we enlisted her neurologist to help with medications for a brief time, and now she needs little pharmaceutical help as long as she adheres to her schedule. She also doesn't work double shifts anymore, nor does she accept working during the hours when her body wants to sleep. She averages about one migraine a month now, which is the lowest frequency she's ever experienced in her life. They usually relate to her menstrual cycle, but she's much more adept at controlling them before they arrive and paying extra special attention to her sleep when she knows she's vulnerable. If there's one thing she does regret, it's not having gotten tuned in to her sleep habits long ago. Having a clear understanding of her boundaries and the role her sleep has in her physical health lets her take total control. *She* runs the show now, not her migraines.

NIGHT 15: PINPOINT YOUR BEST SET OF RELAXATION TECHNIQUES

You might already have a clue as to which relaxation techniques work for you. Maybe you've even managed to come up with some of your own. If you're still struggling, however, do this simple exercise.

First, average two scores from Days 1–4 from your sleep diary in two areas:

1. quality of sleep felt upon awakening
2. feeling refreshed the next day

This allows you to have a baseline of sleep quality and feelings of being refreshed before you try each technique. Input those averages in the charts below (under "Baseline") and then compare those values to the rating you gave on certain days when you tried one of the various techniques. (This should all be recorded in your diary; you simply need to transfer those numbers here.) You'll then be able to identify clearly which had the biggest effect on you.

Reflection and Meditation

	Baseline	Day 2	Day 9	Change
Quality				
Refreshed				

Worry Journal

	Baseline	Day 3	Day 10	Change
Quality				
Refreshed				

Light Reading

	Baseline	Day 4	Day 11	Change
Quality				
Refreshed				

Herbal Tea

	Baseline	Day 6	Day 13	Change
Quality				
Refreshed				

Relaxation CD

	Baseline	Day 7	Day 14	Change
Quality				
Refreshed				

Don't be surprised if the changes noted are small; remember you are likely sleep deprived and still trying to catch up on sleep. Any positive change is good. If you see that in some cases your ratings went up and then down, go back to the schedule for that night and see what you did. How could this have affected your sleep?

It's worth ranking your techniques in order of effectiveness so you know which ones to resort to first, second, and so on.

By now you should be getting into the groove of a good night's sleep. Here are the ten most important reminders of what you should be thinking about daily:

1. Exercise at the right time for your body, at least three times per week.
2. Step down your caffeine consumption in the afternoon.
3. Watch consumption of digestive-unfriendly foods at dinner.
4. Get ready for bed one hour before your self-prescribed bedtime.
5. Have clean bedclothes on and get comfortable.
6. Have a small snack if needed.
7. The bedroom should be cleared of clutter and the following items should have been purchased and installed at the absolute minimum:
   a. 40-watt bulbs
   b. earplugs or a sound machine/MP3 music player
   c. eye shades, blackout shades (drape clips, if needed)
   d. night-lights in strategic places
   e. mattress rotated and new pillows purchased
   f. The temperature should be between sixty-five and seventy-two degrees Fahrenheit (more toward sixty-five, unless you like it warm), with 65 percent humidity.
8. Your bedtime routine should not be taking much longer than sixty minutes.
   a. This routine should include:
      i. thirty minutes of mindless household chores.
      ii. fifteen minutes of hygiene.
      iii. fifteen minutes of relaxation.
   b. Your relaxation technique should be the one that showed you the most change between the quality and refreshed ratings from your average of Days 1 to 4 to the night after the chosen technique
9. Lights-out on time!
10. Wake up on time!

Reminders:
- Do not forget to do your deep-breathing exercises and your Sun Salutes in the morning.
- Did you get your dose of sunlight today?
- Did you take your multivitamin today?

> **Avoid watching TV*, eating, and discussing emotional issues in bed.** The bed should be used for sleep and sex only. If not, you can end up associating the bed with distracting activities that could make it difficult for you to fall asleep.
>
> *Note: If the television has a calming effect on you, then you get a free pass to use it as part of your Power-Down Hour, but be sure to set your TV timer.

NIGHTS 16–21: REVISIT WORRY JOURNAL

Continue to be extremely aware of the ten reminders described in Night 15 for the next six days. These days will help you make up some of that sleep debt that you've been carrying around for so long. Continue to use your sleep diary to take notes and see if your quality ratings and feelings of being refreshed are increasing.

This is the week you should be solidifying your routine and your body should be getting used to your new routine. Also use this week for final tweaking in any areas you feel are not working for you and your sound sleep.

> ### Action Reminder
>
> Have you been using your worry journal? So many of my patients express how useful it is writing down their worries and any unfinished business they might have at the end of the day (as reminders for the next day) that I always press upon new patients the need to start one: *"I can't forget to do ____ tomorrow. I have to remember to take care of ____ tomorrow. I'm so worried about ____ ."*
>
> Try splitting each page of your worry journal into two columns. In the left column, write down the worries that come to you right away, and in the right, come up with a solution for that problem. So in the end you

will have a page that contains your "worries" as well as your To Dos. Then, as you close your journal for the night, you close your worries for the night.

The Sky Is Falling! The Sky Is Falling!

It's 1:45 in the morning, and you've been staring at the ceiling since 10:00 P.M. Thoughts of work and feelings of anxiety keep piling up, and you can't turn your mind off. Just when you think you're about to fall asleep, a new thought charges in and alerts you to wakefulness again. You think, When is it going to end? How am I ever going to get to sleep?

Then, the dread of getting through tomorrow without adequate sleep adds more misery and anxiety to your current situation.

If this sounds familiar, you're among millions of others who experience this routine night after night. They've become so frustrated by their nightly insomnia that the mere awareness of their insomnia (i.e., worrying about not going to sleep) fuels their problem further like a vicious cycle that feeds itself. Remember when I asked you in an earlier chapter whether or not your bedroom conjures feelings of restfulness and peace? If you answered no because the moment you step into your bedroom your mind flashes back to the previous night of restlessness, then cognitive behavioral therapy might be for you. If your bedroom makes you anxious because it reminds you of those troubling moments when you're trying to fall asleep, it's time to rethink *how you think*.

This isn't a new lesson for you. One of the goals of my program has been to change the way you approach and think about sleep. Sleep for most is a perception. There is no way to wake up and say, "Hey I slept about an 8 last night and I feel great," or "Darn, I slept a 3 last night and I feel lousy." My recommendations for setting up your room, preparing for bed, setting aside that Power-Down Hour, and really making an effort to calm your mind through light stretching and relaxation or meditation techniques should go a long way toward shifting how your brain operates when you slip into bed. The worry journal, for example, is an excellent way to train your mind to release itself from stressful, worrisome thoughts. And as you can imagine, stress and anxiety are the leading causes of sleep-onset insomnia in people.

Ask yourself, if you were to take your biggest worries that keep you up at night and assess them *the next morning or afternoon*, would you find them as "big" as you did at bedtime? The same goes for what you might have said to yourself when you couldn't fall asleep quickly. For example, let's assume last night you repeated, "If I don't get to sleep, tomorrow is ruined. I'll suffer enormous consequences. I'm never going to get to sleep . . ." over and over again as you lay awake. Well, what would you think of those statements *today*? Is your day totally ruined? A lost cause? Did you really *never* get to sleep? Maybe, but I don't think so.

Many people distort their worries at bedtime, overexaggerating the magnitude of their woes and the urgency with which they need to remedy them. They also have a tendency to think irrationally as their anxieties rush over them in bed and provoke catastrophic thinking. You might find it helpful to look back through your worry journal and see where you, too, have been a victim of this very human reaction. Highlight thoughts you wrote down that appear absurdly blown out of proportion or just plain silly. This helps you see that many worries are really not that big of a deal, and shouldn't be such huge intruders when it comes to sleep. The reason this happens is quite simple: What else do you have to think about but your worries right before bed? During the day, other activities will likely distract the majority of your worries, so you don't concentrate on them, which is a good thing!

Take a look at Mary's worry journal entry on the next page. This is a fictitious example based on what I've seen in patients. Read her worries in the left-hand column and what she plans to do to conquer them (sometime in the future, not tonight) in the right-hand column. It's easy to see what Mary would be thinking about as she tries to go to sleep. She is worried about her job, about money, about being over-scheduled. She's put her own worries about herself—wanting to lose ten pounds—last, which is typical of those who have a hard time prioritizing themselves first. The emotional issues she's dealing with, namely a "mad" boss and feeling "guilty" for not accepting the role as a volunteer at her daughter's school, are probably riding heavily on her conscience. But if I were to highlight what I think she's exaggerated, I'd point to those emotional worries. Is her boss really that mad at her? Why does she have to feel guilty about saying no to something someone else can—and wants—to do? Likewise, why can't she say no to dinner with friends and take a rain check? What's the big deal? Is it the end of the world? No!

The next time your mind begins to go down that ridiculous route, you can mentally inject a Stop sign and begin to change your thought—and behavioral—process. This wonderful little technique is called cognitive behavioral therapy (CBT), and if you can get good at it, you can reflexively turn negative, insomnia-sustaining thoughts into positive ones that promote sleep.

Mary's Worry Journal

Entry on June 22

1. forgot to make appointment for dog grooming & Anna's pediatric visit	1. make appointments
	   a. forgot (!): write thank-you to Danielle
	   b. Forgot (!): order b-day cake for Aidan

2. boss is mad at me, need to ask for a raise; must reevaluate finances	2. think about what you'd like to ask or ($), and write out what you want to say or write to boss
3. don't want to do dinner Friday night with the Martels—but don't have the heart to back out	3. cancel dinner plans—blame too much going on
4. feel guilty about not volunteering at kindergarten next year	4. ?
5. really need to work out more, I'm ten pounds up	5. figure out times to hit the gym three days this week—tell Steve to take care of kids, stop eating after 7 P.M.

IT'S MORE ABOUT HOW YOU THINK THAN ANYTHING ELSE

Studies have shown that cognitive behavioral therapy, in fact, beats sleeping pills. This proves just how powerful thoughts can be, and that getting restful sleep is more about how you teach your mind to think than using any external trick such as a drug or other sleep aid. So, what is CBT? As its name implies, CBT is one part cognitive and one part behavioral. The cognitive portion of CBT is about recognizing, challenging, and changing the ways of thinking that keep you from falling asleep. If you can't get to sleep easily at night and find yourself tossing and turning while awash in irritating thoughts, chances are you're fueling your own fire with a distorted, stress-inducing behavior. In other words, your worries are minor but are getting too much attention. If you could counter those negative thoughts with a positive one related to the problem, the worry would disappear. Learning how to find those positive thoughts that replace the negative ones and ultimately beat down the stress (thus opening the door for sleep to enter) is what CBT therapists do. They provide information that you can then use to rationalize through your anxiety quickly and get to sleep. Throughout this book I've been helping you with a mild form of CBT by knocking down commonly perceived myths. I've taken those thoughts about sleep and presented real objective data that you may not have known, and with the hope that you begin to change some of your thoughts.

What's most interesting (and a red flag) about people who suffer from chronic insomnia is that their perceptions of their own sleep are not accurate. Just like they distort the importance of their worries right at bedtime, they also distort how well or how bad they are sleeping. Someone who claims she didn't get to sleep until 3 A.M. probably slept a lot more than she thought she did. The proof is in the lab; I've had patients who say they "never slept last night" whose lab results show they slept four or five hours. Eliminating this distortion and snuffing out the fire of negative thoughts is the goal of CBT for sleep.

CBT is also about behavior, which I've already covered at length throughout the book. This is the sleep hygiene part—the ways in which you prepare yourself for sleep. You want to go to bed at the perfect time for your body, and be ready to fall asleep within twenty to thirty minutes. If you're still watching the ceiling thirty minutes later, you should get out of bed and do something that makes you drowsy, such as reading something dull and boring. Lying in bed awake can only add to that fire of anxiety.

CBT is a specific set of processes that require several sessions with a Behavioral Sleep Specialist. Within the American Academy of Sleep Medicine is a select group of individuals who have taken the test to become board-certified in Behavioral Sleep Medicine. Refer to Appendix B for more information. If after you have completed my program you feel as though you have a formal sleep disorder of insomnia, do not panic. A sleep specialist can help you proceed to the next step.

Week 4: Final Phase

Use this week to continue practicing your good sleep habits and testing new methods you haven't yet tried. If, for example, you've been flakey about devoting fifteen minutes to stretching and relaxation just before bedtime, make an effort this week to complete a full fifteen minutes each night and let go of your need to do one more work-related task before your Power-Down Hour. Focus on giving yourself permission to treat that Power-Down Hour as a sacred time.

At this point you should have done some cleaning up of your sleep habits, and have experienced some relief. If you still haven't had much luck in meeting your expectations for sound sleep, it may be time to look more seriously at other sources of sleep problems such as medicines, underlying medical conditions, a true sleep disorder, and your commitment to the outlined recommendations I've already given thus far.

HIDDEN STIMULANTS

If you haven't taken an inventory of your medicine and kitchen cabinets and gotten face-to-face with ingredient labels, now's the time to do so. Victims of powerful marketing and advertising machines, we've become accustomed to popping pills and downing potions that are touted to make us feel and look younger—from diet pills and energy drinks to supplements and vitamin complexes that can contain added ingredients you don't necessarily need and that have a direct impact on sleep. Unless you know what's in your over-the-counter and prescription medicines, including herbal remedies and treatments, you may be consuming stimulants unbeknownst to you.

Because the list of brand names of products that contain hidden stimulants is long and constantly changing, I won't catalog them all here. I urge you, however, to make a list of what pills and supplements you take and either discuss your sleep problems with your doctor, or start by consulting with your pharmacist. Find out what's in your daily doses and learn how to find alternatives that lack stimulants. The word *insomnia* is frequently overlooked on the long list of side effects given for drugs and supplements.

Stimulants are commonly found in medicines to treat headaches, migraines, congestion, asthma, colds, and sinus infections. In recent years, the weight-loss, diet, and supplement industry has been under fire for its sale of ephedra-based products that act as adrenaline-like stimulants. Ephedra is a shrub-like plant found in desert regions in central Asia and other parts of the world. The dried greens of the plant are used medicinally; ephedra's main active medical ingredients are the alkaloids ephedrine and pseudoephedrine, which are the most commonly found ingredients in over-the-counter treatments for respiratory ailments like asthma, and symptoms of colds and sinusitis. They've also been widely used for weight loss, as an energy booster, and to enhance athletic performance. These products often contain other stimulants, such as caffeine or guarana, which consequently increase the potency of the product as well as its potential for adverse effects.

In 2004, the FDA banned the use of ephedrine alkaloids in dietary supplements because of the risk they pose, as they increase the risk of heart attack and stroke. The rule applies to all dietary supplements that contain a source of ephedrine alkaloids, such as ephedra, ma huang, *Sida cordifolia*, and *Pinellia*. But that doesn't mean you can't find this ingredient in other products, such as foods, teas, and medicines.

> Products that are marketed for appetite suppression, weight-loss, metabolic enhancement, increased exercise tolerance, bodybuilding effects, euphoria, increased energy or wakefulness, or other stimulant effects may contain ephedra/ephedrine that will work against you at night.

Herbs or plants that contain the chemical constituent ephedrine include:

- ephedra (also called ma huang, its Chinese name): *Ephedra sinica*
- other Ephedra species such as: *Ephedra shennungiana, Ephedra gerardiana, Ephedra equisetina, Ephedra intermedia*
- *Sida cordifolia*

Herbs or plants that contain caffeine:

- coffee
- green tea—*Camellia sinensis*
- guarana—*Paullinea cupana*
- Maté—*Ilex paraguariensis*
- cola nut (kola nut)—*Cola nitida*, (also other species such as C. *acuminata*, C. *verticillata*, C. *anomala*)

Taking Stock: Examples of common drugs—whether prescribed or over-the-counter—that can trigger sleep problems. (Note that this is a general list, as each brand of drugs will be different. I am not suggesting you avoid these if they've been prescribed or recommended to you by your doctor. I just want you to be aware of them and see if they are having any effects on you.):

- diet and weight-loss pills
- headache and migraine medicines
- painkillers
- antidepressants
- tranquilizers
- drugs for high blood pressure
- cholesterol-lowering drugs (e.g., statins)
- respiratory-treatment drugs (e.g., drugs for asthma, allergies, colds, flus, sinus infections)
- steroids
- thyroid-treatment drugs
- chemotherapy drugs
- anything that claims to give you "energy"

Also think about drug interactions. Don't hesitate to speak with your doctor about the contents of your medicines, and how they all work in combination. If you've got several doctors treating you for various ailments, be sure you keep them apprised of everything you take, whether it's a prescription drug, an over-the-counter drug, or even a supplement you think is harmless. For example, theophylline is yet another ingredient found in drugs that treat respiratory diseases, and it comes under a variety of brand names. Theophylline bears a structural and pharmacological similarity to caffeine. It's also naturally found in black tea and green tea. Common bronchodilating drugs, which open up airways in people with conditions like asthma, often include ephedrine, aminophylline, or norepinephrine—all of which can be very stimulating.

Of all the possible "hidden" ingredients, caffeine is probably the biggest one you'll encounter in unlikely places. For example, Excedrin ("the headache medicine") owes much of its power to caffeine, which acts as a vasoconstrictor. Prescription drugs to treat migraines often also contain caffeine. "Non-drowsy" is sometimes a code word for "stimulating." In the beverage industry, caffeine has been snuck into juice blends and even water bottles so they can be sold as "energy" drinks. Some of these "energy" drinks can contain more caffeine than a cup of strong coffee. Blending with copious amounts of sugar makes for quite a powerful punch. Be particularly wary of "herbal" caffeine drinks that include guarana seeds, kola nuts, and yerba maté leaves. Even though they're natural products, they will keep you feeling perky.

Bottom line: Read your labels and, when in doubt, speak with your doctor or pharmacist. I know those package inserts you find in boxes of medicines can be extremely hard to read. Your best bet is to speak with a professional who's skilled in these meds. The lesson here is to know exactly what you're taking, which you should be doing, anyhow, regardless of sleep problems. I'm not recommending that you do or do not use these products. Just be aware of which ones can be affecting your sleep.

HIDDEN SIDE EFFECTS

If you've been suffering from a chronic illness for which you take regular medicine, it might not be possible to avoid the side effects of your meds. It also might not be possible to make the side effects of your condition, which often bite into a good night's sleep, go away completely. Many patients of chronic illnesses have to live with less-than-perfect sleep. But don't let that fact prevent you from doing your best to get the most out of your sleep and investigating new ways to support a healthy sleep-wake cycle. New drugs with fewer side effects hit the market every day. The combination of sleep aids with your medications might also be a necessary step toward achieving better sleep. These are options you should discuss with your doctor. The point is this: Don't accept poor sleep as an inevitable consequence to your condition. Be open and direct with your doctor. Experiment with new treatments and explore other therapies that might help your sleep coexist with your condition.

I say some of the side effects to your medical condition and its meds are "hidden" because too few people discuss their sleep habits with their doctor. The medical condition steals the attention, and side effects like insomnia, frequent wakenings, and low-quality sleep—whereby no matter how long you sleep, you always wake up feeling tired and not restored—become low-priority. Sleep is such a vital sign of good health that I urge you to make it a priority regardless of your medical condition(s). Be proactive. You might find that you can solve most of your sleep problems through a few lifestyle changes in light of your drug regimen.

Lisa's Story

Lisa has fibromyalgia, a syndrome characterized by chronic pain in the muscles and soft tissues of the body. She also suffers from adult ADHD, insomnia, and was enduring a rough patch in her marriage when she came to me. She was referred to me by her rheumatologist, who was treating her fibromyalgia and told her that unless she could get her sleep under control, her pain would be difficult to control and their options were limited. Fibromyalgia has no known cure, and it embodies a complex set of symptoms that occur together but that have no distinctly known cause. As such, it's a condition that must be managed carefully; treatment is typically focused on controlling pain, fatigue, depression, and other symptoms that commonly occur, including sleep problems. I, quite frankly, was not sure I would be able to help Lisa. The stress from her marriage was ongoing; she had tried multiple medications and was having problems keeping her job due to her sleepiness during the day. A lot of specialists run from these types of patients because they can be difficult to treat, with no end in sight to their myriad problems. Some specialists do even worse by giving them hope of a total cure, or a magic bullet. I knew I had to approach this realistically.

When Lisa and I first met, I liked her right away. She had a positive attitude, and was persistent enough to know that someone out there could help her. Fortunately she was one of my last patients of the day, so I had the luxury of extra time to devote to her.

I aimed to keep her expectations realistic. I told her I could not treat her fibro. I explained that my success with people in her condition came from either 1) identifying an underlying sleep disorder that, once treated, would help ease and control their pain, or 2) addressing poor sleep habits in general, and by following my recommendations, they'd achieve better sleep about 50 percent of the time, which would then help with pain management.

In Lisa's case, we put her on a sleep medication and went to work on determining what factors we could control. Lisa was a candidate for prescription sleep aids because upon monitoring her sleep in the lab, we found that she didn't get adequate deep sleep and experienced a lot of light sleep with frequent arousals. The sleep medication helped her sleep through the night, which was good. But unfortunately it didn't change the quality of her sleep, so she still woke up not feeling totally restored. Due to her fibromyalgia, her chronic pain kept her from getting the best possible sleep.

We then worked backward from her pain, trying to figure out what factors in her life were contributing the most to her pain levels. With chronic conditions like fibromyalgia, the body is under constant physical stress that infringes upon one's ability to achieve perfect, restorative sleep. Ironically, we concluded that stress—of a non-physical nature— was having more of a say in her pain than anything else. In other words, emotional and mental stress were robbing her of a body that could better handle its physical stresses and, in turn, the pain.

Attacking the stress came with practicing relaxation and meditation techniques, plus being super vigilant of her need for that Power-Down Hour. Lisa also got a new job that had more flexible hours and less responsibility. She is now a single mom and reports that the lifestyle changes she made have had a huge impact on her pain management.

HIDDEN SLEEPERS

It wouldn't be fair to point out all the hidden stimulants without doing justice to the hidden sleep promoters. On sight, a sleep aid is usually more obvious than a stimulant. Tylenol PM, for example, is an over-the-counter painkiller that is supposed to be taken at night (hence, "PM"). In addition to the acetaminophen to relieve pain, it contains the drug diphenhydramine (the same active ingredient as in Benadryl), an antihistamine that can induce sleep. Side effects to many of the drugs listed in the "Taking Stock" box, in fact, can impact sleep *on either end of the spectrum*—either inhibiting or promoting sleep, depending on their exact ingredients. For example, painkillers and headache medicines can include stimulants *or* sleep promoters. Cold and allergy medications (whether they are "day" or "nighttime" formulas) can contain stimulants and/or sleepers. As such, the following list of potential sleep inducers isn't so different from what I've already said to watch out for:

- cold and allergy medications that contain antihistamines (these are usually labeled as "nighttime" formulas)
- cough suppressants
- antidepressants
- alcohol
- antihistamines
- sedatives, tranquilizers
- anxiety and antipanic medicines
- seizure medicines
- antipsychotics
- heart medications
- muscle relaxants
- menstrual pain and PMS relief
- pain relievers
- some herbs, naturopathic and homeopathic remedies or supplements (check labeling)
- anything that says "Use caution when driving, operating machinery, or performing other hazardous activities"; likewise, anything that says "May cause drowsiness." (Duh!)

The number of prescription drugs available that can cause drowsiness is colossal. Ask your doctor or pharmacist for specifics on what you take. The people who fall asleep at the wheel aren't just the overtired ones. Many have taken medications that have made them drowsy.

The most important thing to realize is that everyone responds differently to drugs. What makes one person sleepy might make you feel stimulated and alert. And what might put you quickly to sleep might have the opposite effect on your sibling or spouse. The key is knowing how *you* respond so you can make better decisions about what you take and when. In Chapter 11 I'll go into the details of sleep aids, from over-the-counter varieties to prescription drugs. Even sleep aids can cause different reactions in different people.

FOCUSES FOR THE WEEK

To help you finish off your 28-night program, use the following outline to remain focused each day of this final week. Pay particular attention to areas where you know you're weak.

Night 22: Take the next two days off the program. Go back to your old ways and see what kind of rest you get: miss your bedtime, drink as much coffee and alcohol as you want, include foods that will give you acid reflux—anything that you used to do before starting this program. Remember to record in your diary how you feel the next day: refreshed, relaxed, alert in the morning?

Night 23: Keep up the bad habits; I want you to really remember how it used to be.

Night 24: If you've had enough, go back to your new lifestyle and remember how good it feels to sleep again.

Night 25: Are you back to following your bedtime routine? Are you scheduled to sleep in your "Sleep Zone"?

Night 26: Have you been good about the food you are eating and drinking? Remember, these are lifestyle guidelines for a better night's rest. Is your bed partner doing anything to continue to disrupt your sleep? If yes, it's time to have a serious talk.

Night 27: Are you remembering to do your relaxation exercises during your Power-Down Hour? Which ones are you using? (Relaxation recap: Relaxed Standing Forward Bend; the Point-to-Point Release; Cobbler's Pose with Head Rolls; Deep Breathing; the Cat Stretch; the Sponge; and the Relaxation Pose.)

Night 28: How does your bedroom make you feel now? Do you still associate it with feelings of frustration and anxiety because of your experience with sleeplessness? Continue to work toward creating that ideal setting and shifting your mindset so your bedroom conjures nothing but blissful thoughts of rest and relaxation.

Help! A Program Is Not Enough

Sometimes a program is not enough. Sometimes you can't just follow a day-by-day plan and emerge a new person at the other end. Sometimes circumstances prevent you from stopping to follow a regimented course of action. No, I'm not talking about life in general. I'm talking about occupational hazards. If you're a shift worker, constant business traveler, or have odd working hours due to your job, you require special attention. I'll address your needs in the next chapter. I'll also cover other hazards to sound sleep, like vacationing, severe changes in weather, altitude, holidays, and so on. Even when you're not in the comforts of home or on a regular schedule, you don't have to sacrifice a good night's sleep!

I'll answer your most popular questions when it comes to using sleeping aids, pills, and melatonin. There's a reason I've left this topic until last. Find out why.

SoundSleepSolutions.com

Don't forget to check out my Web site at www.soundsleepsolutions.com. There, you can write to me about your personal experiences with sleep, share your own tips on an active message board, and ask questions. I'll post the most frequently asked questions with their answers and possible solutions. Your questions will contribute to an online and active Troubleshooting Guide.

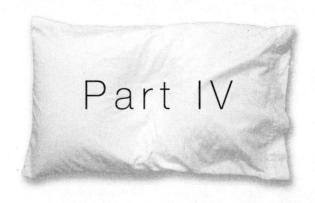

Part IV

The Sleep Aid Industry

CHAPTER 11

What You Want to Know about Pills, Sleep Aids, and Other Potential Hazards to Sound Sleep

You might be surprised that I've hardly touched upon prescription sleeping pills and over-the-counter aids that help you fall asleep faster, stay asleep without interruptions, and wake up feeling refreshed. I also haven't said much about melatonin or various herbs that you can readily buy and that are also supposed to help you sleep better. The point of this book has been to show you ways to achieve sound sleep *without the use of medications*, including over-the-counter (OTC) and prescription drugs. Doctors and patients alike can too easily turn to sleeping pills without first taking an honest look at the patient's lifestyle to see what's really hurting his or her ability to get a good night's sleep.

> You know there's no such thing as a quick fix to weight loss through a diet pill. The same holds true for curing sleep problems and routinely getting a good night's rest. You have to work at it, being mindful of your lifestyle and how it affects your sleep. Be open to trial and error. You'd be amazed by how much a healthy diet and exercise can work wonders on sleep—not to mention your waistline.

Most physicians, unless they have done a great deal of homework, have not been trained in or really know and understand the power of alternative therapies for sleep other than traditional medicines. By resorting to sleeping pills, people risk entering a cycle of depending upon them—even though the latest drugs are not habit-forming. As I

explained in Chapter 10, recent research has shown that cognitive behavioral therapy can be just as effective and last longer for treatment of
insomnia. True, it takes longer to see results, but the solution can last a
lifetime. And it's a completely natural approach.

I encourage physicians to rethink reaching for the prescription pad as
soon as a patient complains, "Hey, Doc, I really don't sleep that well.
Can you give me something?" If the current numbers are accurate,
which indicate that 43 million sleeping-pill prescriptions were written
by U.S. doctors in 2005 (the most recent figures as of this writing), some
docs could be overprescribing meds when in fact they should be looking
at combination therapies to help their patients identify and treat the
underlying root cause of the sleep problem.

> The number of adults ages twenty to forty-four using sleeping pills doubled
> from 2000 to 2004, and the number of kids ages ten to nineteen who take
> prescription sleep remedies jumped by 85 percent during the same period.
> About 11 percent of people admit to using alcohol to help them fall asleep.

I've recommended to and advised physicians that many of their patients try sleeping pills. I don't reject prescription sleep medication entirely. Quite the contrary, recommending these medications to patients
is very much a part of our clinic, and I have professional consulting relationships with some of their manufacturers. These companies are very
interested in how their meds can best be used and in understanding
what the research says about insomnia and poor sleep. But I only suggest
them for specific instances. Like in a lot of other situations in life, there
are appropriate and inappropriate times for their use, be it short term or
long term. I prefer, however, to exhaust all other options first. In fact, in
some cases I recommend medication in conjunction with my program,
which can be very effective.

In this chapter, I dispel some common myths about sleep aids and give
you the guidance you need for determining whether or not you should seek
a doctor's opinion on using a medication. In the later part of the chapter
I'll go into how to handle the most difficult situations when it comes to
getting a good night's rest. I'll also provide a few more tips for traveling, especially if you want to do the 28-night program while on the road.

A New Era of Sleep Medication

Chances are you've noticed the recent blitz in sleep medication ad campaigns as drug companies target consumers directly through radio, print, and the television. It's not without reason, however. First, pharmaceuticals for sleep have been revolutionized in the last decade, and a new generation of sleep medications offer more effectiveness with fewer, less risky side effects or interactions. With any medication, though, everyone responds differently, and there will always be potential side effects. As I write this, reports of bizarre, albeit rare, side effects to one popular brand have surfaced, such as "unconscious" binge eating, driving, and Internet shopping after taking the sleep aid. These people have no recollection of their strange behavior. The people complaining of such experiences reflect less than 1 percent of the total users, and incorrect usage of the drug can be partly to blame. Many of these people have overdosed on the drug, or mixed it with alcohol. Remember to read the package insert; in some cases these effects may already be documented. When used appropriately, however, and always under the supervision of a physician, sleep medications are safe and effective.

More over-the-counter sleep aids are purchased than any other OTC drug, and 25 percent of Americans take some type of medication every year to help them sleep. Benadryl, Nytol, Sominex, Tylenol PM, and Nyquil are popular OTC brands; their main ingredient is an antihistamine called diphenhydramine and, in some cases, alcohol. Ambien, Ambien CR, Lunesta, Rozerem, Indeplon, and Sonata are popular prescription drugs that target specific receptors in the brain, thus setting in motion the sleep process (each of these seems to target different receptors). However, these are not the only class of medications that can be used. Many physicians will try the benzodiazepine hypnotic category, including: Halcion, Dalmane, Restoril, and others. In addition, I've seen physicians use medications that were not originally created as sleep aids but have sleepiness as a side effect, notably Desyrel (Trazodone), Effexor, Amitryptyline, Seroquel, and others. Sometimes minor tranquilizers are prescribed, such as Valium, Librium, Xanax, and Tranxene. *Any medication* can have potential side effects. You should know there is no such thing as a wonder drug for sleep. For a breakdown of common meds used for sleep, see the chart that follows.

Second, our hectic 24/7 society automatically creates a huge market of sleep-deprived people and those who will do anything to maximize their productivity. Many think that if they sleep less, but achieve deeper sleep, then they will be more productive during the day. This may be true, but there are few studies to show that any sleep aid actually increases deep sleep. Most make you fall asleep and stay asleep, but none have been shown to actually increase the kind of sleep that makes you feel refreshed and restored. Nevertheless, there are many who believe that a sleeping pill will cure all of their problems. Just like there are those who believe a diet pill will cure all of their weight problems.

Popular Sleep Aids

Trade or Brand Name	Generic Name or Main Ingredient
Over-the-Counter:	
Benadryl	diphenhydramine
Nytol	diphenhydramine
Sominex	diphenhydramine
Tylenol PM	diphenhydramine
Advil PM	diphenhydramine
Nyquil	doxylamine and alcohol
Prescription:	
Ambien	zolpidem tartrate
Lunesta	eszopiclone
Rozerem	ramelteon
Sonata	zaleplon
Hypnotics	
Halcion	triazolam
Dalmane	flurazepam
Restoril	temazepam
Antidepressants/Antipsychotics	
Desyrel	trazodone
Effexor	venlafaxine
Elavil	amitriptyline
Endep	amitriptyline
Vanatrip	amitriptyline
Seroquel	quetiapine

Trade or Brand Name	Generic Name or Main Ingredient
Benzodiazepines	
Valium	diazepam
Librium	chlordiazepoxide
Xanax	alprazolam
Tranxene	clorazepate

Fact: In a recent State of the Science conference, researchers from around the world concluded that there's not sufficient clinical evidence to support the claims of most OTC medications for sleep. Herein lies an interesting situation where the science may or may not have caught up to the anecdotal evidence based on people's experience. Many OTCs make people feel "fuzzy headed," which is technically not sleepiness but rather a form of relaxation that can easily be mistaken for sleepiness. Therefore, my patients report that these OTCs make them sleep. Some do experience the opposite response, feeling jittery and unable to sleep after taking such an aid. What I often tell people is this: If used as directed and with a physician's review, OTC sleep aids may help relax you enough to go to sleep, but there is no clear clinical evidence that proves these medications increase the likelihood of people falling and staying asleep.

As I already pointed out, there is a time and a place for sleep aids—both prescription and over-the-counter. They come in handy when there is an acute crisis, a sudden stressful event, periods of grief or pain (physical or emotional), or a serious change in schedule. The majority of people will not need these medications for a long time, and those who do often have other underlying medical conditions. People who self-medicate with over-the-counter drugs and without the advice of their doctor can set themselves up for long-term problems. Over-the-counter sleep aids are intended to manage an occasional sleepless night, not chronic insomnia or some other sleep disorder, which could signal a serious underlying problem.

In fact, many of today's prescription sleep aids are safer than OTC sleep aids, especially for older people. Non-narcotic and designed to specifically target receptor sites in the brain that induce sleep, today's class of drugs for sleep ends the days when you could overdose on sleeping pills and never wake up again (as dramatized so many times in the movies).

The problem with many OTC pills is they contain ingredients you may not need, such as painkillers and decongestants or antihistamines—more work for your liver. You also risk waking up with feelings of grogginess or being hung over. What's more, some people can experience a greater alertness instead of sleepiness from OTC medications. (Prescription sleeping pills can also rouse some people instead of promote sleep, so it's not a guarantee. If you're a candidate for prescription sleeping pills, you and your physician may have to try a few to find the one that works best for you.)

This book has not been intended as a treatment for those of you who may suffer from a formal sleep disorder. The purpose of this book has been to help those with *disordered sleep*. If you have a sleep disorder, prescription medications may be quite effective when taken under the guidance of a doctor.

So where do I stand on OTC sleep aids? For occasional use, they are fine, but they are not a long-term solution. What do I consider to be long term? Anything more than one week (seven days). Also, a large note of caution: Just because it's over-the-counter does not always mean it is safe. If one pill worked for a few nights and then stopped, don't up your dose to two, three, or four pills. This may sound a bit strange, but at least once every few months I get a question on WebMD.com from someone asking if it's okay to take a *box* of something a night. No, it's not okay.

Q. Do sleep aids have addictive potential?

A. Yes and no, depending on which medication you are taking. For example, the drug class of benzodiazepines has known addictive properties. But what's often more of an issue is the *psychological* addiction that sleep aids can cause. Addiction as defined medically can mean a series of physiological issues from tremors and vomiting, to insomnia and lethargy. But let's say I'm in a clinic where a patient who hasn't slept well in ten years has been given a nonaddictive medication. He then gets a great night's sleep. Guess what he's going to want again that next night? That pill. And he didn't have to change anything in his life to achieve that great sleep. All he had to do was swallow a pill.

Sleep aids can indeed temporarily fix a problem. Or fix a temporary problem. Does a sleeping pill fix the reason behind poor sleep? Usually not. What it does is mask the real reason for the problem. At times it can give people a false sense of hope and not really go after the root of the issue. Sleeping pills can be an effective component in the treatment of sleep problems, but they aren't the only component in complex problems.

Q. How safe are sleep aids to use long term?

A. This is a very controversial area that not everyone agrees upon. I've seen patients who maintain a sleep-friendly lifestyle but continue to have problems. They follow this entire program to the letter, and their sleep gets better, but for whatever reason it's still not enough. For a few people, long-term use of a sleep aid is okay. Most of the newer sleep medications (those within the last five to ten years) are medications that can be effective long term when used at a steady dosage. In fact, some medications now have long-term indications for use. The older medications, however, are what concern me because taking them in larger doses can be dangerous. One might feel that "one pill is good, but two is better," and it can then be a very slippery downward slope. Whether a person is on an old or a newer type of sleep aid, I always encourage that person to never change dosage without the consent of the doctor, and to always request the lowest possible effective dosage. But to answer the question, can people safely and effectively use sleep aids for a long period of time, the answer is yes.

WHAT ABOUT MELATONIN?

This OTC product continues to get a lot of attention. Many supplement companies and health food stores will tout that melatonin is a "natural" sleeping aid or nightcap because it "naturally" helps regulate sleep-wake cycles. Given the availability of this supplement today, you'd presume it's safe and effective. It's true that melatonin is a hormone your body produces to help it regulate your sleep-wake cycles, but taking additional melatonin in the form of a supplement isn't as good of an idea as you might think without the guidance of a professional. And it's not a regulated drug under the FDA. No other hormone is available in the United States without a prescription. For example, in Europe, melatonin is only available by prescription.

> **Q.** Is melatonin safe to take every night?
> **A.** Again, I go back to the reason why you are having problems sleeping. It is highly unlikely that you have a melatonin deficiency. Melatonin, like anything else, can only be considered a temporary Band-Aid while looking for the root of the problem. If taken properly, meaning at the right dosage and right time, it can be quite effective. But just like long-term use of sleep aids, it must be monitored.

When the sun sets and darkness sweeps over, a pea-size structure located deep between the hemispheres of your brain called the pineal gland secretes this hormone. This usually happens around 9 p.m. Varying patterns of light and dark outside the body control the gland, with environmental information reaching the gland via nerve impulses. As you can imagine, it all starts with the eyes registering either the fall of day or the dawn of another. When wavelengths of light, either from the sun or a bulb, hit the photoreceptors in the back of the eye, signals go directly to your brain's master clock. This master clock is how your brain resets your body daily, by tracking the strength of those signals. In the absence of light, nerve impulses from the eyes are decreased, and secretion of melatonin increases. When melatonin levels in the blood rise, you begin to feel less alert and sleep becomes more inviting. Melatonin levels stay elevated for about twelve hours, falling back to low daytime levels by about 9 a.m. Daytime levels of melatonin are barely detectable.

Melatonin secretion is believed to be involved in the regulation of your twenty-four-hour circadian rhythm; it's how your body and brain learn that it's dark outside. For some animals, this triggers an alerting response while in others, including humans, this normally triggers a sleep-inducing response.

The role of the pineal gland in humans is less well-understood than other glands. Some researchers believe that mood swings are linked to abnormal melatonin secretion patterns. Those who suffer from seasonal affective disorder (SAD), which we'll cover below, might be able to blame their condition on a poorly functioning pineal gland that's thrown off by abnormal and inconsistent light/dark cycles. More recently, melatonin has been linked to cancer (see below).

Generally speaking, melatonin slows body functions, lowers blood pressure and, in turn, core body temperature. When light decreases melatonin production in your body, your brain sends messages for the body to release cortisol and other hormones, which raise blood pressure and core body temperature.

The precise mechanism of melatonin secretion is not well-known. We do know, however, that melatonin isn't just about sleep-wake cycles. It's been shown to help regulate the female reproductive cycle and may also control the onset of puberty. Children who take melatonin can suffer a delay in sexual development. (So never, ever give a child a melatonin supplement.) Furthermore, studies have pointed to melatonin's role in regulating blood flow, specifically in constricting coronary arteries. And it's been suggested that it can increase depression in people prone to the illness.

A hormone with all of these possible effects—even though it's "natural"—isn't something you should be taking without the specific recommendation of a doctor. But even that can be tricky, as most doctors are not familiar with current melatonin research and may not be able to give advice. Moreover, most commercial products are offered at dosages that cause melatonin levels in the blood to rise to much higher levels than are naturally produced in the body. So taking a typical dose (1 to 3 mg) may elevate your blood melatonin levels up to twenty times their normal state. If you take it at the wrong time of day, you may reset your biological clock in an undesirable direction. How much to take, when to take it, and melatonin's effectiveness, if any, for particular sleep disorders are only beginning to be understood. Many more studies need to be performed on this hormone before any sound recommendations—either for or against it—can be made. In the future, we may find several useful applications of melatonin. Right now the data suggests that when used appropriately it can be an effective treatment for transient (short-term) sleeplessness (e.g., jet lag). With correct dosages and a doctor's approval, it can be safe.

If you've been given the green light to use melatonin by your doctor (assuming he or she is experienced with this supplement), then use it as directed to relieve occasional trouble with sleep.

Naturally Calibrating an Upset Body Clock

If you can't go to sleep at night, expose yourself to bright light for ten to fifteen minutes in the morning by either using a light box or, better yet, by going outside. You get bonus points for adding an activity such as walking.

If you wake up too early in the morning, expose yourself to bright light later in the day and go to bed later. If you do this over the course of several days, you should be able to reset your body clock.

If it's dark or dawn when you leave for work and dark or dusk when you head toward home, make an effort to get outside at midday to soak in some of that natural light. You get bonus points again for adding a walk to that mid-day break.

At the root of why melatonin has been aggressively advertised is the sad reality that many people's body clocks *are*, in fact, thrown off course. Why? We don't get enough "sun-time," or exposure to natural light. We shy away from going outside because so much of our lives depends upon indoor activities—on work, the television, the computer, the telephone, the general obligations and choices we make in keeping up with modern life. We continue to gravitate toward a twenty-four-hour indoor lifestyle. If we made a conscious effort to schedule in exposure to natural light during the day, we might have an easier time controlling our biological rhythms . . . and improving our moods.

Q. I sleep a lot more during the winter months and have a harder time feeling motivated in general. What's going on?

A. If you live in an area characterized by lots of overcast, gloomy days in the winter months, you may be a victim of seasonal affective disorder, or SAD, a mood disorder associated with episodes of depression and related to seasonal variations of light. Symptoms of SAD include exhaustion and chronic sleepiness, the need to sleep nine or more hours a night, feelings of sadness, excessive eating and weight gain, and powerful carbohydrate cravings, especially for sugary and/or starchy foods. You might also have a difficult time concentrating. Often these symptoms emerge during the fall and winter months as the days grow shorter and darker, and light becomes an infrequent visitor. They then disappear as spring turns over a new leaf on the day and longer, brighter days herald the onset of summer, which invigorates people's zest for life again and squelches any signs of depression.

Because our internal clocks, rhythms, and regulators are heavily influenced by exposure to light, it's no surprise that one of the main causes of SAD is prolonged deprivation of adequate sunlight that our bodies need to stay on track. The hormones that affect mood, energy, and even food cravings can become imbalanced. Hence, the ways to prevent and/or treat SAD include arranging for exposure to light every day (natural sunlight, or using light box therapy), staying active and maintaining routine physical exercise, and scheduling a mid-winter vacation where you go to a warm, sunny place.

Beware: A full discussion on SAD is beyond the scope of this book, and the techniques herein are not intended to be a treatment for SAD. SAD is a serious problem that requires the attention of a seasoned (no pun intended) professional.

CAN THE MIDNIGHT SNACK IN THE KITCHEN KILL YOU?

While on the topic of melatonin and the body's need for definite cycles of light and dark, it's worth noting startling new research that links exposure to light at night to cancer. The idea of this association started when Eva Schernhammer, M.D., noticed that two of her colleagues—healthy women in their thirties—developed cancer with no risk factors or a history of the disease. Dr. Schernhammer worked rotating night shifts in a cancer ward in Vienna, Austria, from 1992 to 1999. She had to pull ten all-nighters a month in addition to her regular hours. When she landed at Harvard Medical School three years later, she curiously tapped into medical, work, and lifestyle records of nearly 79,000 nurses and discovered that nurses who'd worked thirty or more years on night shifts had a 36 percent higher rate of breast cancer, compared with those who'd worked only day shifts. She continued to uncover more unsettling news, and by late 2005 she had published reports that her fellow female night owls exhibited a 48 percent rise in breast cancer. Women who are blind, on the other hand, had a 50 percent *reduced* risk of breast cancer, compared with their seeing counterparts.

These findings suggest that exposure to light at night may raise the risk of several types of cancer—not just breast. It also shows the profound impact that light can have on our systems, notably our ability to fight diseases like cancer. And light from a buzzing fluorescent bulb in an office or a hospital isn't the only guilty party; working on the computer, watching TV, or even reading under a bright lamp late at night might be enough to alter the biomechanics of your body.

The connection is explained by understanding that melatonin appears to have powerful anti-cancer capabilities. All cells—including cancerous cells—have receptors that bind to melatonin. When a melatonin molecule binds to a breast cancer cell, it counteracts estrogen's tendency to activate cell growth. Recall that melatonin affects reproductive hormones, which might explain why it appears to protect against cancers related to the reproductive cycle—ovarian, endometrial, breast, and testicular. Another feature of melatonin's cancer-fighting strength is its ability to boost the body's production of immune cells that specifically target cancer cells.

Dr. Schernhammer's studies, published in the *Journal of the National Cancer Institute* (2001), provide the first evidence that light can be a risk factor for cancer . . . and that there's a biological relationship between an imbalanced circadian rhythm and cancer. This surely puts a new spin on the idea of getting up for a "midnight snack" and flipping on those bright kitchen lights or opening the fridge to scan what's available. Not to mention the possible weight consequences!

Just ten minutes of light is enough to suppress melatonin in some people. If you have to get up in the night, keep the lights dim. Try and use your night-lights only.

Melatonin's possible influence on immunity and, specifically, cancer cells, however, doesn't make an argument for taking melatonin supplements. It merely reinforces the importance of maintaining a normal circadian rhythm with natural exposure to corresponding light and dark cycles so your body can produce the perfect amount of melatonin for its needs. An excessive or scarce amount of this hormone will work against you.

Q. Is it ever okay to keep a small stock of sleeping pills in the medicine chest *just in case*? And if so, do I go for an over-the-counter aid, or should I ask my doctor to write me a prescription for emergencies?

A. Sleeping pills should be something you genuinely need, meaning they should not be something that you ask your doctor for "just in case." You wouldn't ask your doctor for painkillers to keep "just in case," would you? Probably (hopefully) not. But if you and your doctor feel that you have a legitimate reason for the use of sleep aids, then by all means you should have them.

Q. Is it ever okay to use alcohol as a nightcap?

A. Alcohol will help you fall asleep, but it will interrupt the quality of your sleep. Instead of using alcohol as a nightcap, try some herbal tea and a warm bath.

Herbal Supplements

The question about herbal treatments for sleep comes my way constantly. Are all herbal remedies safe and effective? Of course, the answers vary depending on the herb in question. Here is a brief overview of the more popular herbs touted for sleep:

Valerian: Valerian extract from the root has been widely used around the world since the seventeenth century, and is especially popular in Europe for its sedative effects. These effects are attributed to benzodiazepine-like activity (meaning it affects the same receptor sites), which is how hypnotic drugs act on the brain. Most of the studies on valerian have been on individuals with sleep disorders and healthy volunteers, and several experiments do consistently indicate that valerian extract may decrease the time it takes to fall asleep, as well as enhance the quality of that sleep by increasing deep sleep. Common names for valerian include baldrian, radix valerianae, and Indian valerian. It appears to be effective in both fresh/dried form and as a liquid extract.

German chamomile: Not to be confused with Roman chamomile (both from the daisy family), German chamomile has mild sedative effects similar to valerian and is most often found in teas. If you're allergic to daisies, however, you might want to avoid this one. In addition, anyone allergic to ragweed, asters, or other members of this family or individuals taking anticoagulant medications should steer clear of chamomile.

Kava: Kava (also known as kava-kava) appears to act as a depressant on the central nervous system, and has been reported to be a muscle relaxant and analgesic. Three studies have found sleep-promoting effects of kava, but mostly on anxiety-related sleep problems. It should not be used in conjunction with alprazolam. Heavy use can cause visual disturbances.

Lavender: Usually studied as lavender oil, it is reported to have depressant effects on the central nervous system and musculature. Subjects in one study who were given three minutes of aromatherapy with lavender oil reported relaxation, less depression, and increased cognitive skills. Its sedative qualities are not well-tested. However, of the research collected, lavender has been shown to be comparable to hypnotics. More research is under way.

As you can tell, we don't know everything when it comes to these herbs. You'll find them in many tea concoctions, or sometimes as supplements in tablet form. Others you'll encounter that are marketed to help you sleep include primrose, fennel, Jamaica dogwood, California poppy, St. John's wort, lime blossom, hops, passionflower, rosemary, and skullcap. This list goes on and on. In *The Review of Natural Products*, Fourth Edition, there are forty-two herbals listed under "sedatives" and sixteen under "sleep disorders."

If you're going to try any one or combination of these, do some research into the pros and cons, especially considering your current drug regimen. I would never recommend using any of these while taking another medication, as they could have unknown side effects. Interactions between over-the-counter herbs and prescription drugs happen frequently. People over the age of fifty with chronic conditions for which they require long-term drug therapy need to be extra cautious. The enzymatic processes in the body that metabolize prescription drugs are the same that metabolize other foreign compounds, including all-natural herbs and OTC medicines. Using medicinals simultaneously always has a potential for adverse interactions.

If you do try an herbal remedy and have a poor reaction, immediately contact your physician and let him or her know what is going on. Finally, as I have said numerous times, evaluate your reasons for taking something and try to determine if you can make a lifestyle change first before resorting to such treatments.

The Five Guidelines to Using a Sleep Aid

1. Think of sleep aids as remedies of last resort, *unless* you have a medical condition that causes your sleep problems and your use will continue only through the treatment of that medical condition.

2. Think of sleep aids as remedies of last resort, *unless* insomnia or some other sleep problem is a side effect of a medication you are taking to treat a medical condition. Medications for depression, for example, can cause sleep disturbances, so your doctor may also want to prescribe a sleep aid.

3. Sleep aids can be used in conjunction with my program to break the cycle of insomnia, but sleep aids should not be used for the long term.

4. If you're among the approximately 10 percent of people who have chronic insomnia, you may require a sleep aid for long-term use.

5. When taking a sleep aid of any kind for short-term situations, remember to avoid driving or making big decisions. See if you can tough it out without having to use the sleep aid.

Sleepless in Shift Work

If Dr. Schernhammer's research makes you queasy because you do have to work odd hours and accept a less-than-optimal light-dark rhythm, don't overreact and let this news ruin your day. Just because you're a shift worker who spends a lot of time under artificial light in the wee hours of morning doesn't mean you have an inescapable death sentence. Not by a long shot. A quarter of the workforce does shift work, so you're not alone and you can still make your health and wellness a priority despite your work obligations.

I've left the subject of shift work to this last chapter because it's beyond the scope of this book. Dealing with shift work deserves its own tome. In fact, there are entire businesses that focus solely on the shift worker. I'll provide a few quick tips, but recommend that if you fall into this category, refer to Appendix B for Web resources and recommended literature that can help you with this unique situation.

> Shift work is working in blocks of time periods that typically rotate in eight-hour "shifts" around a twenty-four-hour clock. Generally speaking, the morning shift is 8 A.M. to 4 P.M.; the evening shift is 4 P.M. to midnight; and the "graveyard" shift is midnight to 8 A.M. (there are some variations on this framework). In many companies that operate twenty-four-hour facilities, employees work one shift for a few days or weeks, then take on a new shift so everyone gets to cover the different types of shifts over that twenty-four-hour period.

While it's possible for a shift worker to become totally adjusted and biologically aligned with any single shift, be it the regular day shift or the graveyard shift, most shift workers are at the mercy of rotating shifts that disrupt their rhythms. Or they break their rhythms on the weekends or on days off when they finally get a chance to catch up with their families. Shift workers typically have two hours less sleep than other workers and, as a result, they have more problems with diabetes, psychological problems, divorce, and all kinds of health problems.

It's not easy being a shift worker, and the older you are, the harder it may be to maintain such work without suffering increasing bouts with insomnia as the body's adapting abilities decline with age. But there's good news: Being a mindful shift worker who respects your sleep time as much as your work and family time can have an enormous impact on your quality of life, on the balance you can create, and on your overall satisfaction with work and home life.

To attempt my 28-night program, simply adjust your Night 1

experiment for the shift change. Here are a few things you'll want to try to keep in mind:

- If your shifts have to rotate, request that they rotate clockwise—from day to night to graveyard—instead of the reverse. It's much easier to adapt to a clockwise rotation than a counterclockwise one, which, unfortunately, is how many places conduct shift work. Also, ask your employer if you can keep the same shift for two weeks at a time before rotating. This will give you an opportunity to try to determine your Sleep Zone.
- Schedule your sleep time and set strict rules for making sure you get your Zs during that time period. Turn off your phones, televisions, and don't respond to anyone unless it's an emergency.
- Sleep in your bedroom (not on the living room couch) and make sure you have the right setting. It should be dark and free of distractions and noise.
- Be very careful about alcohol, caffeine, and nicotine use. Review my rules, as these substances can have a greater effect on you.
- Watch what you eat toward the end of your shift, in preparation for sleep. Remember that after your shift, you should not just rush home to bed. When you were on a day shift, you likely never did that, either. You'd go home, relax, have dinner, etc. Many shift workers try to rush home in the dark to catch some sleep, but this can incite more problems with sleep.
- Form a support group out of your own family. Tell them your needs and be attentive to their needs as well.

Again, refer to Appendix B for more resources.

On the Road with Your 28-Night Program

Dealing with jet lag is very similar to what shift workers experience when they have to adjust to a new "time zone"—that of their new shift. The internal biological rhythm gets thrown for a spin, and it takes time for the body to adapt. Alertness Solutions, a consulting firm headed by Mark Rosekind, Ph.D., who is a former director of NASA's Fatigue

Countermeasures Program, conducted a study of travelers on trips crossing more than two time zones and lasting two to four days. The study revealed some interesting findings and confirmed others:

- A few hours of lost sleep combined with business travel significantly reduces performance.
- Business travelers perceived themselves as performing at a much higher level than they actually did (a 20 percent drop).
- Travelers actually performed best during midday, not early morning, which many consider to be prime time for productivity.
- Of those who rated their performance highly, half fell asleep unintentionally on the trip.
- Study participants slept, on average, only five hours the night before a trip—the lowest of the entire seven-day monitoring period. But they reported getting an hour more sleep than they actually did.
- Those who exercised during their trip performed an amazing 61 percent better than non-exercisers.
- Study participants registered a total sleep loss of almost eight hours by the time they returned home, the equivalent of one full night's sleep.

In Chapter 3 we covered a few ideas for managing business trips, especially when you have to cross time zones. You don't have to be a business traveler, however, to heed those recommendations. Any kind of traveling requires special attention to sleep if you expect to look and feel your best. Generally, it takes about one day to adjust for each hour of time change. A trip across one time zone for a couple of days should not cause much of a problem for most people. In general, "losing" time is more difficult to adjust to than "gaining" time. So traveling east is harder on our bodies than traveling west. An "earlier" bedtime may cause difficulty falling asleep and increased wakefulness during the early part of the night. Going west, you're likely to fall asleep easily but may have a difficult time waking. The way I remember it is, "East is least, and west is best."

Attempting the 28-night program on the road presents a few challenges: The principle culprit is jet lag, and the secondary culprit is your environment. You already know your circadian rhythm greatly influences when you sleep, and the quantity and the quality of your sleep. It may also be altered by the timing of various factors, including naps, bedtime, and exercise.

Resetting your internal clock to adapt more quickly to the time changes is the secret to dealing with traveling and warding off jet lag. Your circadian rhythm is internally generated but is influenced by the environment, behavior, and medications. It is important to expose yourself to the light during the waking hours as much as possible and, conversely, do not expose yourself to bright light when it is dark outside. Remember: Even the light from a computer screen or turning the light on in the bathroom in the middle of the night can adversely affect your sleep.

In addition to the tips given in Chapter 3, here are a few more suggestions:

- Plan ahead. Get a good night's sleep the two nights prior to departing. If you have to complete the 28-night program on the road, travel during Week 3, since by then, many of the experiments are complete and your data has been collected.
- Eat healthfully and exercise the day before you leave.
- Dress appropriately. Wear comfortable, warm, loose-fitting, and layered clothing.
  ➤ Consider thick socks or slippers in your on-board sleep kit so you can take off your shoes.
- Bring your travel kit for the journey (see page 276).
- Bring your home-away kit for the destination (see page 275).
- Lower your expectations for having a perfect traveling experience. Remember: It's hardly ever a perfect experience.
- On the plane, drink lots of water—regular, not carbonated—to reduce excess gas.
- On the plane, be mindful of alcohol and caffeine. (One drink in flight equals two on the ground.)
- On the plane, use a decongestant or antihistamine, if necessary, to relieve air pressure. Or, try gum.
- Consider a short nap on a short flight and a longer one on a longer flight. Nap toward the end of flights. Time your naps carefully,

avoiding emerging from one in deep sleep. If you know you're going to touch down at 12:00 P.M., try setting your watch to take a
nap at 11:30. If you're landing at 3:00 P.M. and you're really
sleepy, consider a nap at 1:30.

- Book your hotel room with thought. Consider room location,
amenities, quality of beds, pillows, attention from the front
desk, etc.
- Practice the same bedtime routines as you do at home—defend
your Power-Down Hour even while away. Because you'll likely
not have any chores to do, consider doing some extra relaxation
techniques.
- Get your exercise in each day. Make sure your hotel has a gym, or
you can go for a brisk walk.
- Switch to the new time as soon as you arrive when traveling
west. If you're traveling east and only going to be gone for one to
two days, try staying on your old time zone.
- Eat well. Avoid heavy, fatty meals. Watch excess alcohol and caffeine consumption. If you're going to be entertaining clients,
limit your alcohol to one glass of white wine or a light beer. Remember to drink a full glass of water with it.
- Avoid nicotine close to bedtime, if not entirely.
- Give yourself a day to adjust before having to make critical decisions or engaging in any activity that requires 110 percent of you.
- Don't forget to get your daily dose of bright light.

Sleeping medications can be an effective sleep manager, but they have
no effect on realigning the body's biological imbalance caused by traveling to a different time zone. Also be careful not to take them until you are
in the air. If there are mechanical difficulties and you need to de-plane after taking a sleep aid, it could be difficult.

Switching over to the new time zone will happen quicker if you go to
bed and wake up at your usual time but in this new time zone. That first
night might be hard to get past—you'll either not be ready for bed when
it's time or will have difficulty staying awake depending on whether
you've traveled east or west. On your second day, be sure to get as much

sun or bright light as possible, and preferably early in the morning. That should help reset your clock naturally. If your body wants to sleep but you need to be awake, hit the outdoors and soak in some sunlight. What if it's raining? Find a good source of bright light.

Some people have asked me why they can't just stay on their own time zone. This is a possibility, and it might work if your travels are not lengthy—fewer than two days. But understand that by staying on your own time zone, you'll have a hard time making the most out of your trip. For example, if your usual bedtime is 10 P.M. and you've gone from New York to Los Angeles, you'll have to call it a night in L.A. at 7 P.M. or sooner to get your Power-Down Hour in. And that can be impossible to do, for business travelers and vacationers alike.

Q. I always dread the annual daylight saving change in time. In the spring, when the clocks move forward an hour, I can't get out of bed early enough for several days. Is there a way to "wean" myself off the old time and be ready for the new time when it comes?

A. Yes, actually there is a way. Try moving your bedtime and your wake time by fifteen minutes, beginning four weeks out from the date of daylight saving time. By the time you get to the change in time, you'll already be on the correct time.

The amenities that can make a difference in how well you sleep away from home:

❑ designated quiet areas
❑ soundproof rooms
❑ luxurious bedding and a menu of pillows
❑ earplugs
❑ eye covers
❑ blackout curtains
❑ relaxing, sleep-promoting music
❑ night-lights in room and bathroom
❑ aromatherapy, soaps, oils, and other bathroom pleasures
❑ wake-up calls
❑ an exercise room
❑ a spa facility

If your hotel does not provide you with these types of amenities, that may or may not be a problem. Below I have given you the start of a Traveling Sleep Kit to help in those specific situations that may require just a touch of home.

The Traveling Sleep Kit for the Plane and Hotel

- ❏ C-shaped pillow that fits around your neck
- ❏ your tunes (i.e., iPod or MP3 player) and headphones (consider sound-dampening headphones); relaxation/meditation music
- ❏ sleep diary
- ❏ worry journal (may want to keep a travel-size worry journal)
- ❏ earplugs
- ❏ eye covers
- ❏ bottled water (not carbonated)
- ❏ gum or decongestant
- ❏ energy bar of some sort
- ❏ curtain clip
- ❏ travel alarm
- ❏ aromatherapy
- ❏ a small stash of OTC medications for possible on-the-road illness (e.g., pain reliever like ibuprofen or acetaminophen, and something to relieve gas and constipation)
- ❏ multivitamins

Getting Your Zs While Vacationing

The same recommendations for sound sleep that I've already given work for vacations, too. Prepare for your vacation as you would a serious business trip. Shift over to any new time zone as fast as you can by sticking to your usual bedtimes and wake times *in the new time zone*, and getting a healthy dose of light and activity each day. I can't reiterate enough what a tremendous impact light has on the body's natural recalibrating systems.

Going from sea level to high altitude (more than 5,000 feet), as in taking an alpine ski vacation to the mountains, presents unique problems. Many people suffer from altitude sickness, characterized by headache, stomach upset, loss of appetite, nausea, feelings of weakness, breathlessness, increased heart rate, and fatigue. And as a result of all these physical maladies comes insomnia or waking up feeling ill in the middle of the night. It takes anywhere from one to three days to adjust to a high altitude, but everyone responds differently. Obviously, the higher the altitude, the more your body has to adapt. It has to make some adjustments in order to deal with the lower oxygen content of the air and a lower air pressure. This process, called acclimatization, is slowed down by dehydration, overexertion, alcohol, and other depressants. Depressant drugs include barbiturates, tranquilizers, and yes— even sleeping pills. By taking a sleeping pill, you lengthen the time it takes your body to function comfortably in the altitude, which means your symptoms can worsen and you'll suffer longer.

Combating altitude sickness starts with staying extremely hydrated, avoiding strenuous activity (okay, if you plan on skiing your heart out, go easy that first day; your muscles will thank you, too), and carefully watching your alcohol and nicotine intake, if not abstaining from these entirely. Other tips to try:

- Eat more carbohydrates. Go for getting more than 70 percent of your calories from carbohydrates while in the high country.
- Keep a jug of water by your bedside in case you wake up feeling parched and headachy in the middle of the night.
- Try some antacid pills to help relieve any gastrointestinal problems and excess gas you might be having.
- For a headache—or any aches, for that matter—that you want to treat, be sure to use medications that don't have any added stimulants, such as generic acetaminophen, ibuprofen, or naproxen sodium.
- Use a humidifier. High-altitude usually mean low humidity levels.

The trick to sleeping well while on vacation is in maintaining your normal sleep hygiene habits even though you're away from home. It's natural to live a little differently while vacationing, as many of us stay out later at night or enjoy more cocktails than normal. But that doesn't mean you can't remain vigilant about how your choices affect your sleep, and take some precautions. After all, what good is a vacation if you can't get sound sleep and come back to work feeling refreshed and rejuvenated?

> **Q.** Is it okay to let my body sleep as much as it wants during a vacation? Or will that work against me, so I should keep to the same strict sleeping schedule even though I don't have any serious work or social obligations? In other words, can I let my sleep schedule go?
>
> **A.** If you're terribly sleep deprived and have not begun your 28-night program, then use your vacation as an opportunity to pay back your sleep debt. Get all the sleep you need. However, if you dramatically change your sleep schedule while on vacation, you'll experience sleep deprivation for the first few days back at home due to your new sleep patterns. This is a big reason why so many of us need a vacation from our vacation. The key factor here is to try and continue to maintain your wake time.

Final Note from the Sleep Doctor

By now, I hope you've gained not only a lot of information on ways to improve your sleep, but also a greater appreciation for sleep and its role in your life. Sleep medicine is still in its infancy and every year we uncover new knowledge that confirms what we've all been concluding based on our own experience: that sleep is an essential ingredient in all that we do. I don't doubt that we will ever understand how sleep affects us completely. And we may continue to struggle with a clear understanding of exactly why we sleep and its wondrous responsibility in keeping our bodies maintained, balanced, and healthy. Like the universe itself, the association between sleep and our bodies' machinery might be infinite. My hope is that you begin to seek solutions to chronic problems through better quality and quantity sleep.

I wish you the best of luck in your journey and I encourage you to come back to this book when life derails your healthy sleeping habits and you need to revisit my program.

Sweet dreams,
Dr. Mike, Ph.D.

SoundSleepSolutions.com

Don't forget to check out my Web site at www.soundsleep solutions.com. There you can write to me about your personal experiences with sleep, share your own tips on an active message board, and ask questions. I'll post the most frequently asked questions with their answers and possible solutions. Your questions will contribute to an online and active Troubleshooting Guide.

ACKNOWLEDGMENTS

I owe numerous people many thanks for helping me get to the point in my career where I've been given the privilege to write a book and hopefully help a lot of people. It's hard to know where to start. Forgive me if I miss someone, just know that you are not forgotten.

First, my children, Cooper and Carson. They motivate me to do the best I can. And to Lauren, for putting up with me throughout the whole process.

Next is my father, who simply taught me persistence, and that was all I needed to accomplish this feat.

Dr. Sheldon Solomon, for having the confidence in me to run his research subject, fail miserably, and start my career.

Drs. Dick Bootzin, Mike Perlis, and James Wyatt, for giving me my first job in sleep and my first friends in the sleep medicine world.

Drs. Illeana Arias, Amos Zeichner, and Henry Adams, for believing in me and taking me in when no one else would; for not kicking me out when you could; and giving me a hard enough time to straighten out (Hank, I hope you can read this wherever you are).

Dr. Patrick O'Connor and the entire Department of Sport and Exercise Psychology at the University of Georgia, for letting an outsider in, and teaching me how to understand the research. It's the foundation of everything.

Drs. Jeanetta Rains, Terry Brown, and Howard Roffwarg, for opening my eyes to clinical sleep medicine. I don't think I have blinked yet.

Drs. Tom DeMarini, Marc Pollock, David Snider, Harold Jackson, and the entire crew at Southeastern Lung Care, thanks for my first real job, teaching me day in and out clinical sleep medicine and letting me grow.

Drs. Jeff Michaelson, Rana Rab, and Suzi Ie, thanks for your friendship and patience, and for respecting me when you did not have to.

Lynn Discordia, for being there for me in more ways than I can count.

Dr. Duanne Johnson, thanks for all the mentoring, advice, and love. You are one of the best people I have ever known.

Dr. Stuart Myers, for being one of my closest friends and confidants. You may never know how important your friendship is to me and your belief in our cause is so very important. Thanks also for letting WebMD know about me.

Dr. Russell Rosenberg, Gail Reid, and Terry Malloy, thanks for all of your support for all of my crazy ideas and my first paid speaking engagement. I miss you guys.

Nan Forte, Jennifer Newman, Karoli Kuns, Katie Leopold, and Sandee LaMotte, thanks for believing that sleep medicine was a topic that needed attention and helping establish my credibility.

Kevin Kowalski, Rob Bezner, and everyone at Crowne Plaza Hotels, thanks for giving me a big break. The Sleep Advantage program was and still is the single largest sleep hygiene program ever done. What a great vision.

Marc Fedor, Jyllene Miller, Heather Iorillo, Anthony Bauman, Chuck Ensign, Mike Pierce, and John, thanks for the opportunity.

Jennifer Sind and Jo Coutts, thanks for teaching me something every time we get together.

To everyone at Areté Sleephealth, thanks for putting up with my crazy schedule, my wacky ideas, and making it all fun.

Thanks to all of the sleep technologists I have worked with in Phoenix, Atlanta, and all over the world. I learn something new every time.

Robin Hommel, you are the one who actually set the ball in motion for this book. I will be forever grateful; by the way, Jane should have picked me the first time around.

Erin Saxton and the gang at the Idea Network, what can I say? You are my compass. You could never have a better friend or team member. Allyson, Sue, and Jennifer, you girls bring it to a whole new level.

Bonnie Solow, I feel lucky to have you as my agent, for I know this process would have never happened without your imagination, knowledge, and tenacity. Thanks.

Russ Kamalski, I have tremendous respect for you and all you do for me. Just name it, anytime, anywhere and you got it.

Patty Aubrey, you are an amazing, fun, creative, intelligent person who is helping me change my life. Thanks for seeing my future.

Kristin Loberg, thanks for creeping inside my head and making sense of it all. You are truly gifted and I know we will continue to do great things together and help a lot of people.

Brian Tart and Neil Gordon, thanks for believing in the topic and making this look easy. A big thanks to Dutton for believing in a first-time author. We've got a lot more books to come.

Lisa Johnson and Beth Parker, thanks for working with my team to get the word out.

Bob Keegan, thanks for the photos, friendship, and philosophy.

Thank you to all of my patients, for teaching me about sleep and letting me help.

A special thanks to Adam and Lisa. In a very public way you both have let the world know your issues and it is a better place for it.

APPENDIX A:
SLEEP DIARY

| 1 = poor |
| 10 = great |

Week One

NIGHT 1:
 Wake time (that morning):
 Proposed wake time:
 Planned lights-out time:

MORNING 2:
 Lights-out time (previous night):
 How long you think it took you to fall asleep:
 The time you woke up:
 The quality of your sleep (rate 1–10):
 How refreshed you feel in the a.m. (rate 1–10):

MORNING 3:
 Lights-out time (previous night):
 How long you think it took you to fall asleep:
 The time you woke up:
 The quality of your sleep (rate 1–10):
 How refreshed you feel in the a.m. (rate 1–10):
 Notes on bedtime routine:
  What will you strive to do (or not do) every night in preparation
  for bedtime?

On a scale of 1–10, how relaxed did self-reflection/meditation while lying down make you feel?

Plans for today:
    Caffeine cutoff time:
    Alcohol cutoff time:
    Your last cigarette:

Nighttime exercise:
    List your biggest stressors of the day:
1.
2.
3.
4.
5.

MORNING 4:

    Lights-out time (previous night):
    How long you think it took you to fall asleep:
    The time you woke up:
    The quality of your sleep (rate 1–10):
    How refreshed you feel in the a.m. (rate 1–10):
    On a scale of 1–10, how relaxed did listing out your stressors and their solutions make you feel?
    How much:
        Caffeine you ingested and when:
        Nicotine you ingested and when:
        Alcohol you ingested and when:
    Ask yourself: Should you move your cutoff times back an hour?
    Exercise for the day (see Chapter 8):

Bedroom Plans

Long Term	*Short Term*
_____	_____
_____	_____
_____	_____

_____   _____
_____   _____
_____   _____
_____   _____
_____   _____

MORNING 5:

Lights-out time (previous night):

How long you think it took you to fall asleep:

The time you woke up:

The quality of your sleep (rate 1–10):

How refreshed you feel in the a.m. (rate 1–10):

On a scale of 1–10, how relaxed did reading something light/fun/boring make you feel?

How much:

Caffeine you ingested and when:

Nicotine you ingested and when:

Alcohol you ingested and when:

What's left to do to your room to make it a better sleep environment?

Plans for today:

Which two relaxation techniques will you try tonight?

1.

2.

MORNING 6:

Lights-out time (previous night):

How long you think it took you to fall asleep:

The time you woke up:

The quality of your sleep (rate 1–10):

How refreshed you feel in the a.m. (rate 1–10):

On a scale of 1–10, how relaxed did your bedtime technique make you feel? Which stretches and/or guided imagery ideas did you try?

How much:

Caffeine you ingested and when:

Nicotine you ingested and when:

Alcohol you ingested and when:

What's left to do to your room to make it a better sleep environment? Did you remember (or plan) to do some stretching, such as the Sun Salute, this morning?

Plans for today:
    My food and beverage cutoff time (about four hours before bedtime):

MORNING 7:
    Lights-out time (previous night):
    How long you think it took you to fall asleep:
    The time you woke up:
    The quality of your sleep (rate 1–10):
    How refreshed you feel in the a.m. (rate 1–10):
    On a scale of 1–10, how relaxed did your bedtime technique make you feel? Which stretches and/or guided imagery ideas did you try?
    How much:
        Caffeine you ingested and when:
        Nicotine you ingested and when:
        Alcohol you ingested and when:
    What's left to do to your room to make it a better sleep environment? Did you remember (or plan) to do some stretching, such as the Sun Salute, in the morning?
    What was the time of your last meal? Was it at least four hours before bed?
    What did you eat?
    Have you gone out and bought a good multivitamin?

    Plans for today:
        Time of exercise:
        Resting pulse:
        Pulse after exercise:

MORNING 8:
    Lights-out time (previous night):
    How long you think it took you to fall asleep:
    The time you woke up:
    The quality of your sleep (rate 1–10):

How refreshed you feel in the a.m. (rate 1–10):

On a scale of 1–10 how relaxed did your bedtime technique make you feel? Which stretches and/or guided imagery ideas did you try? How much:

　　Caffeine you ingested and when:

　　Nicotine you ingested and when:

　　Alcohol you ingested and when:

What's left to do to your room to make it a better sleep environment? Did you remember (or plan) to do some stretching, such as the Sun Salute, in the morning?

What was the time of your last meal? Was it at least four hours before bed?

What did you eat?

Did you exercise yesterday? If so, what did you do and when did you do it?

Evaluate the sleep schedule:

Ask yourself:

　　Is my bedtime working for me?

　　Do I feel refreshed in the morning?

　　Should I shift my bedtime back or forward some?

Week Two

Use the following chart in conjunction with the exercises and instructions in Chapter 9 to complete your entries.

Sleep Diary

Date:	Bedtime/ wake time:	Quality/ duration of sleep:	Times awake at night:	Caffeine/ alcohol consumed; when consumed:	Food/ drink:	Emotions/ stress: Relaxation technique:	Drugs/ medication:

Date:	Bedtime/ wake time:	Quality/ duration of sleep:	Times awake at night:	Caffeine/ alcohol consumed; when consumed:	Food/ drink:	Emotions/ stress: Relaxation technique:	Drugs/ medication:

Date:	Bedtime/ wake time:	Quality/ duration of sleep:	Times awake at night:	Caffeine/ alcohol consumed; when consumed:	Food/ drink:	Emotions/ stress: Relaxation technique:	Drugs/ medication:

Date:	Bedtime/ wake time:	Quality/ duration of sleep:	Times awake at night:	Caffeine/ alcohol consumed; when consumed:	Food/ drink:	Emotions/ stress: Relaxation technique:	Drugs/ medication:

Date:	Bedtime/ wake time:	Quality/ duration of sleep:	Times awake at night:	Caffeine/ alcohol consumed; when consumed:	Food/ drink:	Emotions/ stress:	Drugs/ medication:
						Relaxation technique:	

Date:	Bedtime/ wake time:	Quality/ duration of sleep:	Times awake at night:	Caffeine/ alcohol consumed; when consumed:	Food/ drink:	Emotions/ stress:	Drugs/ medication:
						Relaxation technique:	

Date:	Bedtime/ wake time:	Quality/ duration of sleep:	Times awake at night:	Caffeine/ alcohol consumed; when consumed:	Food/ drink:	Emotions/ stress:	Drugs/ medication:
						Relaxation technique:	

Most effective relaxation techniques:

Best time to exercise:

Week Three

Sleep Diary

Date:	Bedtime/ wake time:	Quality/ duration of sleep:	Times awake at night:	Caffeine/ alcohol consumed; when consumed:	Food/ drink:	Emotions/ stress:	Drugs/ medication:
						Relaxation technique:	

Date:	Bedtime/ wake time:	Quality/ duration of sleep:	Times awake at night:	Caffeine/ alcohol consumed; when consumed:	Food/ drink:	Emotions/ stress:	Drugs/ medication:
						Relaxation technique:	

Date:	Bedtime/ wake time:	Quality/ duration of sleep:	Times awake at night:	Caffeine/ alcohol consumed; when consumed:	Food/ drink:	Emotions/ stress:	Drugs/ medication:
						Relaxation technique:	

Date:	Bedtime/ wake time:	Quality/ duration of sleep:	Times awake at night:	Caffeine/ alcohol consumed; when consumed:	Food/ drink:	Emotions/ stress:	Drugs/ medication:
						Relaxation technique:	

Date:	Bedtime/ wake time:	Quality/ duration of sleep:	Times awake at night:	Caffeine/ alcohol consumed; when consumed:	Food/ drink:	Emotions/ stress:	Drugs/ medication:
						Relaxation technique:	

Date:	Bedtime/ wake time:	Quality/ duration of sleep:	Times awake at night:	Caffeine/ alcohol consumed; when consumed:	Food/ drink:	Emotions/ stress:	Drugs/ medication:
						Relaxation technique:	

Date:	Bedtime/ wake time:	Quality/ duration of sleep:	Times awake at night:	Caffeine/ alcohol consumed; when consumed:	Food/ drink:	Emotions/ stress:	Drugs/ medication:
						Relaxation technique:	

Week Four

Sleep Diary

Date:	Bedtime/ wake time:	Quality/ duration of sleep:	Times awake at night:	Caffeine/ alcohol consumed; when consumed:	Food/ drink:	Emotions/ stress:	Drugs/ medication:
						Relaxation technique:	

Date:	Bedtime/ wake time:	Quality/ duration of sleep:	Times awake at night:	Caffeine/ alcohol consumed; when consumed:	Food/ drink:	Emotions/ stress:	Drugs/ medication:
						Relaxation technique:	

Date:	Bedtime/ wake time:	Quality/ duration of sleep:	Times awake at night:	Caffeine/ alcohol consumed; when consumed:	Food/ drink:	Emotions/ stress:	Drugs/ medication:
						Relaxation technique:	

Date:	Bedtime/ wake time:	Quality/ duration of sleep:	Times awake at night:	Caffeine/ alcohol consumed; when consumed:	Food/ drink:	Emotions/ stress:	Drugs/ medication:
						Relaxation technique:	

Date:	Bedtime/ wake time:	Quality/ duration of sleep:	Times awake at night:	Caffeine/ alcohol consumed; when consumed:	Food/ drink:	Emotions/ stress:	Drugs/ medication:
						Relaxation technique:	

Date:	Bedtime/ wake time:	Quality/ duration of sleep:	Times awake at night:	Caffeine/ alcohol consumed; when consumed:	Food/ drink:	Emotions/ stress: Relaxation technique:	Drugs/ medication:

Date:	Bedtime/ wake time:	Quality/ duration of sleep:	Times awake at night:	Caffeine/ alcohol consumed; when consumed:	Food/ drink:	Emotions/ stress: Relaxation technique:	Drugs/ medication:

APPENDIX B: RESOURCES

Web Sites

Consumer Organizations and Foundations

General:

SoundSleepSolutions
This is the company I co-founded with Dr. Stuart Meyers dedicated to raising the awareness of and providing solutions for sleep problems and disorders.
www.soundsleepsolutions.com

National Sleep Foundation
www.sleepfoundation.org

The Better Sleep Council
www.bettersleep.org

National Center on Sleep Disorders Research
www.nhlbi.nih.gov/about/ncsdr

Sleep Home Pages
www.sleephomepages.org

Stanford University Center of Excellence for the Diagnosis and Treatment of Sleep Disorders, Sleep Well
www.stanford.edu/~dement

Sleep Research Society
www.sleepresearchsociety.org

National Heart, Lung and Blood Institute, Sleep Disorders
www.nhlbi.nih.gov/health/public/sleep

American Academy of Sleep Medicine
www.aasmnet.org

Sleep Apnea

American Sleep Apnea Association
www.sleepapnea.org

Narcolepsy

Narcolepsy Network
www.narcolepsynetwork.org

Restless Legs Syndrome

Restless Legs Syndrome Foundation
www.rls.org

Traffic Safety

Victims of Irresponsible Drowsy Drivers
www.voidd.com

Smart Drivers Break for Sleep; Drowsy Driving Basics for College Students : www.drowsydriving.cornell.edu

Professional Sleep Associations and Societies

American Academy of Sleep Medicine (AASM)
www.aasmnet.org

Academy of Dental Sleep Medicine
www.dentalsleepmed.org

National Institutes of Health National Center on Sleep Disorders
Research (NCSDR)
www.nhlbi.nih.gov/about/ncsdr

Society for Light Treatment and Biological Rhythms (SLTBR)
www.sltbr.org

Sleep Research Society (United States) (SRS)
www.sleepresearchsociety.org

Sleep Centers

There are more than 800 accredited sleep centers in the United States.
The most efficient way to find one near you is to go to the site run by
the American Academy of Sleep Medicine at www.sleepcenters.org.
From there, you can click on your state and locate which center is most
convenient for you.

Info for Shift Workers

You'll find a wealth of information dedicated to shift workers on the
Internet. A few examples of resourceful sites are listed below.

Circadian Technologies
www.circadian.com
Although Circadian is a research and consulting firm that helps
companies better manage shift work, you'll find lots of useful
resources such as a newsletter and other publications geared toward
the shift worker and his or her family.

Alert @ Work
www.alertatwork.com

Alertness Solutions
www.alertness-solutions.com

Retail Outlets for Sleep Products

The Litebook Company (light therapy boxes)
www.litebook.com
e-mail: info@litebook.com or sales@litebook.com
phone: 877-723-5483
#6, 941 South Railway St. SE
Medicine Hat, Alberta, Canada
T1A 2W3

Sound Sleep Solutions, Inc.
www.soundsleepsolutions.com
Go here for a variety of self-care products, such as earplugs, white
noise machines, and aromatherapy that you can buy directly
through our link to Amazon.com.

SleepLamps.com
www.sleeplamps.com
e-mail: info@sleeplamps.com
Photonic Developments, LLC
7890 Summerset Drive
Walton Hills, OH 44146

The Ear Plug *Super* Store
http://earplugstore.com
phone: 918-478-5500
P.O. Box 658
Hulbert, OK 74441

Hunter Douglas (window treatments that consider light and sound)
www.hunterdouglas.com
Go to the Web site to find a local dealer.

The Warm Company
www.warmcompany.com (see "Window Treatments" under
"Products")
e-mail: info@warmcompany.com
Use the Web site to locate where to buy its products locally.
phone: 800-234-WARM; 206-320-9276

Marpac Corporation
www.marpac.com (see "Sound Conditioners")
e-mail: info@marpac.com
phone: 800-999-6962
fax: 910-602-1435
P.O. Box 560
Rocky Point, NC 28457

Blooming Grove
www.bloominggrove.com
e-mail: info@bloominggrove.net
phone: 862-368-5877
This company offers excellent bath and linen products.

NOTES

Page 1.

David Lazarus, "Sleep Aids a Booming Business," *San Francisco Chronicle*, March 3, 2006. Statistics about prescriptions written for sleeping aids as well as other drugs, including over-the-counter medicines, can be found at IMS Health, a provider of market intelligence to the pharmaceutical and health-care industries (www.imshealth.com).

Page 7.

National Institutes of Health, Department of Health and Human Services. For more information, visit the NIH's National Heart Lung and Blood Institute at www.nhlbi.gov or contact the NHLBI's Information Center at P.O. Box 30105, Bethesda, MD 20824-0105, or at 301-592-8573 or 240-629-3255 (TTY). The NIH (www.nih.gov) is the medical research agency for the U.S., and includes twenty-seven institutes and centers. It's "the primary federal agency dedicated to conducting and supporting basic, clinical, and translational medical research. It also investigates the causes, treatments, and cures for both common and rare diseases."

Page 11.

The National Sleep Foundation's 2005 "Sleep in America" poll is cited throughout the text. The NSF is, according to its site, "an independent nonprofit organization dedicated to improving public health and safety by achieving understanding of sleep and sleep disorders, and by supporting sleep-related education, research, and advocacy." As part of its continued research, the NSF conducts annual surveys; in 2006, the organization focused on teens and sleep. You can download any of the NSF's findings, as well as access a multitude of information, at its Web site (www.sleepfoundation.org). Or contact the organization directly at 1522 K Street NW, Suite 500, Washington, DC 20005; Ph: (202) 347-3471; Fax: (202) 347-3472.

Page 11.

Daniel Kahneman et al., "A Survey Method for Characterizing Daily Life Experience: The Day Reconstruction Method (DRM)," *Science* (December 3, 2004), vol. 306, no. 5702, pp. 1776–80.

Pages 17–18.

A. Dijksterhuis et al., "On making the right choice: the deliberation-without-attention effect," Comment in *Science* (February 17, 2006), vol. 311, no. 5763, pp. 1005–7. For related articles and experiments, refer to the following citations:

A. Dijksterhuis, "Think different: the merits of unconscious thought in preference development and decision making," *Journal of Personal Social Psychology* (November 2004), vol. 87, no.5, pp. 586–98.

J. D. Schall, "Neural basis of deciding, choosing and acting," *National Review of Neuroscience* (January 2001), vol. 2, no.1, pp. 33–42.

J. A. Debner and L. L. Jacoby, "Unconscious perception: attention, awareness, and control," *Journal of Experimental Psychology: Learning, Memory, and Cognition* (March 1994), vol. 20, no. 2, pp. 304–17.

Page 18.

Dr. Hans P. Van Dongen et al., "The cumulative cost of additional wakefulness: dose-response effects on neurobehavioral functions and sleep physiology from chronic sleep restriction and total sleep deprivation," *Sleep* (March 15, 2003), vol. 26, no. 2, pp. 117–26. For more information, see also: Dr. Hans P. Van Dongen, "Brain activation patterns and individual differences in working memory impairment during sleep deprivation," *Sleep* (April 1, 2005), vol. 28, no. 4, pp. 386–8.

Page 18.

As previously noted, the 2005 "Sleep in America" poll's "Summary of Findings" can be downloaded at www.sleepfoundation.org or obtained by contacting the organization.

For data on general statistics on sleep loss in the U.S., refer to the study released April 4, 2006, by the Institute of Medicine, which is an arm of the National Academy of Sciences. Reported by the Associated Press on April 4, 2006, in "Chronic sleep problems costing U.S. billions: Millions of Americans suffer from insomnia, related disorders, study finds." Retrieved April 21, 2006, at www.msnbc.com. Additionally, for more information on sleep and driving, see the study released April 20, 2006, by the Virginia Tech Transportation Institute for federal safety regulators (and partially funded by the NHTSA, or National Highway Traffic Safety Administration). Reported by Reuters on April 4, 2006, in "Study: Driver drowsiness big safety problem: Tired drivers are four times more likely to crash than rested motorists." Retrieved on April 21, 2006, at www.msnbc.com.

Page 20.

MIT Classics Archive, "On Sleep and Sleeplessness" (or *"De Somno et Vigilia"*) by Aristotle as translated by J. I. Beare. Retrieved January 21, 2006, at http://classics.mit.edu/Aristotle/sleep.html.

Page 21.

Refer to the National Highway Traffic Safety Administration (NHTSA) Web site at www.nhtsa.gov for more information and to download studies and research.

Page 23.

Linda H. Lamb, "Sleep study: To snooze, or to lose? Those who sleep longest found to be more likely to have health problems," *Wilkes Barre Times-Leader,* March 14, 2006. Check out forthcoming studies by Shawn Youngstedt and colleagues at the University of South Carolina's Arnold School of Public Health. Youngstedt's team is testing long sleepers to see whether restricting their sleep time has any ill effects. At this writing, the studies had not yet concluded.

To review the study published in *Cancer Research,* which followed twelve thousand women over twenty years and revealed that those who reported sleeping nine hours or more per night had about one-third the risk of developing breast cancer—compared to women who slept less—refer to the following citation: P. K. Verkasalo et al., "Sleep duration and breast cancer: a prospective cohort study," *Cancer Research* (October 15, 2005), vol. 65, no. 20, pp. 9595–600.

Page 25.

Barbara Kantrowitz, "The Quest for Rest," *Newsweek,* April 24, 2006. Also see cover story "Why Women Can't Sleep" and "To Sleep? That's a Dream," by Allegra Goodman, published in the same magazine. Both retrieved April 20, 2006, on www.msnbc.com.

Pages 34–5.

The statistics on exactly how many people suffer from insomnia are not entirely clear. While it's been reported that about 70 million Americans, or one in three people, suffer from insomnia a few nights a week or more, based on polls like those from the National Sleep Foundation, other studies have reported other numbers. For example, a study released in 2006 by the Institute of Medicine shows that 30 million Americans, more than one in ten, suffer specifically from chronic insomnia. As I note in the text, insomnia is a general term that can cover many troubles related to sleep. In some cases, it's considered a disorder. In others, it's a symptom of something else, such as stress or anxiety. Suffice it to say no matter which study you look at, insomnia is a problem for millions and is by far the leading cause of sleep-related issues.

Page 35.

National Sleep Foundation poll, "Sleep in America," 2005.

Page 38.

These statistics were pulled from a twenty-eight-country survey by ACNielsen, the marketing arm of TV ratings giant Nielsen Media Research. The results were released March 1, 2005, and reported by Jennifer Harper for *The Washington Times,* March 10, 2005 ("Portuguese pull most late nights, sleep poll finds"). You can access several of ACNielsen's reports on their Web site at www.acnielsen.com, and specifically,

"Sleepless in America: 34% in Bed After Midnight, 29% Up by 6 a.m.: ACNielsen Survey Finds Late Bedtime Hours Are Common Around the World." Released April 4, 2005 in a news release out of the company's main office in Schaumburg, IL.

Also refer to: "Sleepless in Asia: 40% of Asia Pacific Consumers Aren't in Bed Until After Midnight." Released February 28, 2005, in a news release from Hong Kong and available for download on ACNielsen's Web site.

For a fascinating look at how people sleep around the world, refer to the following citation:

C. R. Soldatos et al., "How do individuals sleep around the world? Results from a single-day survey in ten countries," *Sleep Medicine* (January 2005), vol. 6, no. 1, pp. 5–13.

Page 48.

A number of scientists have explored the subject of caffeine's effect on athletic performance. Of interest are the following recent studies:

K. T. Schneiker et al., "Effects of caffeine on prolonged intermittent-sprint ability in team-sport athletes," *Medicine and Science in Sports and Exercise* (March 2006), vol. 38, no. 3, pp. 578–85.

G. R. Stuart et al., "Multiple effects of caffeine on simulated high-intensity team-sport performance," *Medicine and Science in Sports and Exercise* (November 2005), vol. 37, no.11, pp. 1998–2005.

C. R. Bruce et al., "Enhancement of 2000-m rowing performance after caffeine ingestion," *Medicine and Science in Sports and Exercise* (November 2000), vol. 32, no. 11, pp. 1958–63.

D. G. Bell and T. M. McLellan, "Effect of repeated caffeine ingestion on repeated exhaustive exercise endurance," *Medicine and Science in Sports and Exercise* (August 2003), vol. 35, no. 8, pp. 1348–54.

Page 68.

National Sleep Foundation recommendations, www.sleepfoundation.org.

Page 69.

For more on Rush University's sleep study, go to www.rush.edu. You should be able to locate its Sleep Disorder Service and Research Center from this site. To contact by phone, call 312-942-5440 or e-mail at contact_rush@rush.edu.

Page 69.

According to *Guinness World Records* in 2000, Melvyn Switzer's record for being the loudest snorer (coming in at 87.5 decibels on June 28, 1984—the level of a fire siren) was broken by Kare Walkert of Kumla, Sweden, who suffers from obstructive sleep apnea. Walkert's snoring level was measured at 93 decibels—the level of a lawn mower—at the Orebro Regional Hospital on May 24, 1993.

Page 93.

R. B. Tofle et al., "Color in Healthcare Environments," The Coalition for Health

Environments Research (CHER), 2004. For more information, go to www.chere search.org.

Page 104.

I credit much of my information on pillows to an interview I conducted with Dan Schecter, Vice President of Sales and Marketing for the Consumer Products Division at Carpenter Company. He explained a lot of the latest technology to me, as well as debunked a few old myths related to the bedding industry.

Page 113.

The fact versus fiction information on mattresses was adapted from an article published by *Consumer Reports* in June 2005. While some of this report came under fire following *CR*'s study, the real fact remains that mattress selection is a personal choice. Only you can decide what's good for your body and sleep. For more evaluations on mattresses by *CR*, go to www.consumerreports.org.

Page 119.

The study of "The Best and Worst Cities for Sleep" was conducted by Bert Sperling's BestPlaces, a research firm in Portland, Oregon, that specializes in studies ranking and rating metropolitan areas in the U.S. This particular study consisted of two main parts. The first identified the ten best and ten worst cities for sleep, and the second part used data provided by the Centers for Disease Control and Prevention (CDC) to analyze the relationship between sleep and different physical and emotional health factors. The primary source of data for the study was the Behavioral Risk Factor Surveillance System (BRFSS). Conducted annually by the CDC, the surveillance system is among the world's largest telephone surveys, querying over 250,000 households about health matters, both physical and emotional. For more information about this study and other "Best and Worst" reports, go to www.best places.net. To see a complete breakdown of this particular study's results city by city plus an overview of how the conclusions were made, go to www.bestplaces.net/docs/ studies/AmbienSleep.aspx.

Pages 123–24.

Studies that demonstrate the link between sleep and the hormones that control appetite—plus the correlation to weight control—have been widely reported. Of interest are the following studies:

K. Spiegel et al., "Leptin levels are dependent on sleep duration: relationships with sympathovagal balance, carbohydrate regulation, cortisol, and thyrotropin," *Journal of Clinical Endocrinology and Metabolism* (November 2004), vol. 89, no. 11, pp. 5762–71.

K. Spiegel, R. Leproult, and E. Van Cauter, ["Impact of sleep debt on physiological rhythms"]. [Article in French], *Revista de Neurologia* (Paris), (November 2003), vol. 159 (11 Suppl), 6S11–20.

K. Spiegel et al., "Brief Communication: Sleep curtailment in healthy young men is associated with decreased leptin levels, elevated ghrelin levels, and increased hunger and appetite," *Annals of Internal Medicine* (December 7, 2004), vol. 141, no.11, pp. 846–50.

G. Copinschi, "Metabolic and endocrine effects of sleep deprivation," *Essential Psychopharmacology* (2005), vol. 6, no. 6, pp. 341–7.

S. Taheri et al., "Short sleep duration is associated with reduced leptin, elevated ghrelin, and increased body mass index," *PLoS Medicine* (December 1, 2004), vol. 3, e62.

Page 124.

Daniel Kahneman et al., "A Survey Method for Characterizing Daily Life Experience: The Day Reconstruction Method (DRM)," *Science* (December 3, 2004), vol. 306, no. 5702, pp. 1776–80.

Page 130:

S. Viner, J. P. Szalai, and V. Hoffstein, "Are history and physical examination a good screening test for sleep apnea?" *Annals of Internal Medicine* (1991), vol. 115, pp. 356–359.

R. J. Davies, N. J. Ali, and J. R. Stradling, "Neck circumference and other clinical features in the diagnosis of the obstructive sleep apnoea syndrome," *Thorax* (1992), vol. 47, pp. 101–105.

C. A. Kushida, B. Efron, and C. Guilleminault, "A predictive morphometric model for the obstructive sleep apnea syndrome," *Annals of Internal Medicine* (1997), vol. 127, pp. 581–87.

Page 131.

J. E. Gangwisch et al., "Inadequate sleep as a risk factor for obesity: analyses of the NHANES I," *Sleep* (October 1, 2005), vol. 28, no. 10, pp. 1217–20.

Page 135.

Studies and polls are routinely done to evaluate the general public's approach to New Year's resolutions, as well as how well those resolutions are sustained. Most recently, in January 2006 Harris Interactive conducted a poll for the Wall Street Journal Online's Health Industry edition. The poll's findings were released January 25, 2006: "New Year's Resolutions: Easier to Make than to Keep; New survey shows U.S. adults struggle with their resolutions to lose weight, get more sleep and stop smoking." For more information, contact Harris Interactive, a market research firm: Info@harrisinteractive.com (www.harrisinteractive.com); 800-866-7655.

Page 136.

T. L. Horvath, and X. B. Gao, "Input organization and plasticity of hypocretin neurons: possible clues to obesity's association with insomnia," *Cell Metabolism* (April 2005), vol. 1, no. 4, pp. 279–86.

Pages 140 and 143.

Jim Horne, *Sleepfaring: The Secrets and Science of a Good Night's Sleep* (New York: Oxford University Press, 2006).

Page 147.

National Sleep Foundation's "Sleep in America" poll, 2004.

Page 149.

The press release that covered this British study was released April 18, 2005, and accessed online at http://www.britishsnoring.co.uk/pdf/nssws.pdf on November 22, 2005. It's cited as follows: "British Snoring & Sleep Apnoea Association questionnaire survey. Snoring affects your love life—true or false" (2005).

Another citation you may want to check out is the following: "Snoring can affect your sex life," by M. Madani; American College of Oral & Maxillofacial Surgeons, May 2001.

Page 151.

For more information about Dr. David Weeks's work and conclusions, refer to *Secrets of the Superyoung: The Scientific Reasons Some People Look Ten Years Younger Than They Really Are—And How You Can, Too* by David Joseph Weeks and Jamie James (New York: Berkley Publishing Group, 1999).

Page 159.

For more information about Dr. Mark Rosekind's work and research, refer to his company's Web site at www.alertness-solutions.com.

To explore the counterintuitive relationship between sleep deprivation and one's ability to perform exercise, refer to the following studies, among others:

J. P. Scott and L. R. McNaughton, "Sleep deprivation, energy expenditure and cardiorespiratory function," *International Journal of Sports Medicine* (August 2004), vol. 25, no. 6, pp. 421–26.

J. P. Scott, L. R. McNaughton, and R. C. Polman, "Effects of sleep deprivation and exercise on cognitive, motor performance and mood," *Physiology and Behavior* (February 28, 2006), vol. 87, no. 2, pp. 396–408.

M. J. Plyley et al., "Sleep deprivation and cardiorespiratory function. Influence of intermittent submaximal exercise," *European Journal of Applied Physiology Occupational Physiology* (1987), vol. 56, no. 3, pp. 338–44.

D. W. Hill et al., "Aerobic and anaerobic contributions to exhaustive high-intensity exercise after sleep deprivation," *Journal of Sports Science* (October 1994), vol. 12, no. 5, pp. 455–61.

Pages 163–64.

Dr. Sara C. Mednick, who holds a Ph.D. in psychology, specializes in sleep research with a focus on napping. At this writing, she is a research scientist at the Salk Institute for Biological Studies in La Jolla, California. She has completed numerous studies, however, with other institutions and has been widely published. For more information about her work and studies, refer to her Web site at www.saramednick.com. Her studies of interest include:

S. C. Mednick, A. C. Arman, and G. M. Boynton, "The time course and specificity of perceptual deterioration," *Proceedings of the National Academy of Sciences of the United States of America* (March 8, 2005), vol. 102, no. 10, pp. 3881–5.

S. C. Mednick and Sean P. A. Drummond, "Sleep: a prescription for insight?" *INSOM* (Summer 2004), no. 3.

S. C. Mednick, Ken Nakayama, and Robert Stickgold, "Sleep-Dependent Learning: a nap is as good as a night," *Natural Neuroscience* (July 2003), vol. 6, no. 7, pp. 697–8.

S. C. Mednick et al., "The restorative effect of naps on perceptual deterioration," *Natural Neuroscience* (July 2002), vol. 5, no. 7, pp. 677–81.

Page 241.

The research to support the value of cognitive behavioral therapy (CBT) in treating sleep problems, notably insomnia, is plentiful. Articles and studies of note for further information include:

C. M. Morin, "Cognitive-behavioral approaches to the treatment of insomnia," *Journal of Clinical Psychiatry* (2004), vol. 65 (Suppl), no. 16, pp. 33–40.

J. D. Edinger and M. K. Means, "Cognitive-behavioral therapy for primary insomnia," *Clinical Psychology Review* (2005), vol., 25, no. 5, pp. 539–58.

M. T. Smith and D. N. Neubauer, "Cognitive behavior therapy for chronic insomnia," Clinical Cornerstone (2003), vol. 5, no. 3, pp. 28–40.

M. T. Smith and M. L. Perlis, "Who is a candidate for cognitive-behavioral therapy for insomnia?" *Health Psychology* (2006), vol. 25, no. 1, pp. 15–9.

J. Backhaus, F. Hohagen, U. Voderholzer, and D. Riemann, "Long-term effectiveness of a short-term cognitive-behavioral group treatment for primary insomnia," *European Archives of Psychiatry and Clinical Neuroscience* (2001), vol. 251, no. 1, pp. 35–41.

Page 256.

While 11 percent of adults report using alcohol to fall asleep, according to the National Sleep Foundation's poll in 2005, it's possible that 11 percent is an extremely conservative number, and that many more do resort to alcohol for purposes of getting to sleep. The percentage of shift workers, for example, is closer to double the average—at 22 percent.

Pages 265–66.

Eva S. Schernhammer et al., "Night work and risk of breast cancer," *Epidemiology* (January 2006), vol. 17, no. 1, pp. 108–11.

Eva S. Schernhammer et al., "Rotating night shifts and risk of breast cancer in women participating in the nurses' health study," *Journal of the National Cancer Institute* (October 17, 2001), vol. 93, no. 20, pp. 1563–68.

Eva S. Schernhammer et al., "Night-shift work and risk of colorectal cancer in the nurses' health study," *Journal of the National Cancer Institute* (June 4, 2003), vol. 95, no. 11, pp. 825–8.

Eva S. Schernhammer et al., "Epidemiology of urinary melatonin in women and its relation to other hormones and night work," *Cancer Epidemiology Biomarkers and Prevention* (June 2004), vol. 13, no. 6, pp. 936–43.

S. Davis, D. K. Mirick, and R. G. Stevens, "Night shift work, light at night, and risk of breast cancer," *Journal of the National Cancer Institute* (October 17, 2001), vol. 93, no. 20, pp. 1557–62.

Page 268.

The Review of Natural Products, 4th Edition, Edited by Ara Dermarderosian, Lawrence Liberti, and John A. Beutler (Lippincott Williams & Wilkins, 2005).

Pages 269–70.

The topic of shift work, while beyond the scope of this book, is a subject all on its own. Refer to Appendix B for a list of resources you can use to find more information about dealing with shift work.

Page 272.

For more on Dr. Mark Rosekind's work and research, go to his company's Web site at www.alertness-solutions.com. The site contains a lot of useful resources and information.

INDEX

ABOUT THE AUTHOR

Michael Breus is a practicing Ph.D. in clinical psychology with a specialty in clinical sleep disorders. He oversees nine sleep labs across Southern California and Arizona as the senior vice president of clinical operations of Areté Sleephealth. In addition to treating patients and training other sleep doctors, he consults with major airlines and hotel chains to provide effective sleep tips for their customers. Dr. Breus is the designated health expert on WebMD.com for sleep and writes the column *Sleep Matters* for the new WebMD magazine. He lives in Scottsdale, Arizona, with his wife and two children.

Thank you for your dedication to getting a good night's sleep.
For more information, please visit www.yoursleepcoach.com.